'This book not only enriches and  potential of art therapy in the Eas insights from the very sources of mz practices already fully or partially ad.....by western professionals. *Art Therapy in Asia* may become Asia's most valuable healing export to the world. I hope it is translated into all languages for doctors, teachers, and therapists of all disciplines."

—*Bobbi Stoll, founder of the International Networking Group of Art Therapists (ING/AT) and Past President of the American Art Therapy Association (AATA), currently chair of the International Member Subcommittee of the AATA, Los Angeles, USA*

"*Art Therapy in Asia* is an ambitious project in which a dedicated group of art therapists has participated, each participant bringing his or her own interest and specialism to the task. The thematic organisation of the book enables the reader to focus on the similarities and differences in approach to art therapy across the enormously wide range of cultures, languages, religions, and values that make up 'Asia'."

—*Professor Diane Waller, OBE, MA, DPhil, Dip Group Psych, FRSA, Emeritus Professor of Art Psychotherapy, Honorary Visiting Professor, Centre for Mental Health, Imperial College London, and Principal Research Fellow, School of Applied Social Science, University of Brighton, UK*

"*Art Therapy in Asia* offers the reader a clearly articulated, richly textured picture of the theoretical, cultural, spiritual, and political forces at play in the work of Asian art therapists. Uniquely Eastern in perspective, it also elucidates the common ground between East and West and makes a significant and timely contribution to the increasingly global practice of art therapy."

—*Catherine Hyland Moon, author of* Studio Art Therapy: Cultivating the Artist Identity in the Art Therapist *and editor of* Materials and Media in Art Therapy: Critical Understandings of Diverse Artistic Vocabularies, *Associate Professor, Art Therapy Department, School of the Art Institute of Chicago, USA*

"This book is an important departure from previously published literature on art therapy: it sensitively and constructively challenges euro-centric assumptions about health, identity, and spirituality and it also offers some very good practical advice on the practice of art therapy in Asia. It therefore provides a great contemporary overview of this topic and describes an inspiring way to think about ethnicity, culture, and healing that many art therapists will find helpful. Its relevance goes much further than Asia and it should be widely read worldwide."

—*Val Huet, Chief Executive Officer, British Association of Art Therapists*

"Although I've visited and taught art therapy in Korea, Japan, Taiwan, China, India, and Thailand, this book opened my eyes and expanded my mind in breathtaking ways. I hope that all Western art therapists will read and learn from this thoughtful, stimulating contribution to the global growth of art therapy."

—*Judith A. Rubin, Ph.D., ATR-BC, Department of Psychiatry, University of Pittsburgh, President of Expressive Media Inc. and Past President and Honorary Life Member of the American Art Therapy Association, USA*

"The lovely metaphor and question is the essence of the book. Is art therapy in Asia steeped to the bone in the cultures of the East, or do we know it is Asian by the merest touch of silk? The book shows both of these to be part of the answer. Kalmanowitz, Potash, and Chan have gathered chapters from art therapists working in ten regions across Asia and the results are inspiring. They show the potential for adapting art therapy for different places and people in the world. They give touching insight into different Asian practice, and they show how things shared are helpful for practice everywhere."

—*Chris Wood, author of* Navigating Art Therapy: A Therapist's Companion *and Director of Art Therapy Northern Programme, Sheffield, UK*

Art Therapy in Asia

of related interest

Art Therapy and Postmodernism
Creative Healing Through a Prism
Edited by Helene Burt
Foreword by Joy Schaverien
ISBN 978 1 84905 253 5
eISBN 978 0 85700 536 6

Focusing-Oriented Art Therapy
Accessing the Body's Wisdom and Creative Intelligence
Laury Rappaport
ISBN 978 1 84310 760 6
eISBN 978 1 84642 852 4

Art in Action
Expressive Arts Therapy and Social Change
Ellen G. Levine and Stephen K. Levine
Foreword by Michelle LeBaron
ISBN 978 1 84905 820 9
eISBN 978 0 85700 270 9

Spirituality and Art Therapy
Living the Connection
Edited by Mimi Farrelly-Hansen
Foreword by Deborah Bowman
ISBN 978 1 85302 952 3
eISBN 978 1 84642 219 5

Art Therapy Techniques and Applications
Susan I. Buchalter
ISBN 978 1 84905 806 3
eISBN 978 1 84642 219 5

Art Therapy in Asia

To the Bone or Wrapped in Silk

*Edited by Debra Kalmanowitz,
Jordan S. Potash and Siu Mei Chan*

Forewords by Shaun McNiff and William Fan

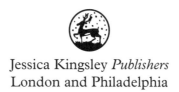

Jessica Kingsley *Publishers*
London and Philadelphia

Fig. 21.1 from Pollock and Van Reken 2001 on p.295 is reproduced by permission of Piyachat Ruengvishesh Finney

First published in 2012
by Jessica Kingsley Publishers
116 Pentonville Road
London N1 9JB, UK
and
400 Market Street, Suite 400
Philadelphia, PA 19106, USA

www.jkp.com

Library of Congress Cataloging in Publication Data
Art therapy in Asia : to the bone or wrapped in silk / edited by Debra Kalmanowitz, Jordan S. Potash, and Siu Mei Chan ; forewords by Shaun McNiff and William Fan.
     p. cm.
  Includes bibliographical references and index.
  ISBN 978-1-84905-210-8 (alk. paper)
  1. Art therapy--Asia. 2. Asians--Counseling of. 3. Asians--Mental
health. 4. Psychotherapy--Cross-cultural studies. I. Kalmanowitz,
Debra, 1965- II. Potash, Jordan S. III. Chan, Siu Mei.
  RC489.A7A7695 2012
  616.89'1656--dc23
                                    2011046142

British Library Cataloguing in Publication Data
A CIP catalogue record for this book is available from the British Library

ISBN 978 1 84905 210 8
eISBN 978 0 85700 449 9

Printed and bound in Great Britain

Contents

Figures and tables

Acknowledgements

We would like to thank the clients and workshop participants throughout Asia who helped to prompt the new strategies and creative ways of working described in this book; our colleagues in Asia and around the globe who contributed, and continue to contribute, to the discovery of meaningful and culturally relevant theories and practices; and our families and friends who supported us in this endeavour.

Foreword

Shaun McNiff

Art Therapy in Asia makes a world statement about the art therapy process, furthering application to the majority of the people on earth,[1] and arguably doing even more for art therapy by offering in-depth reflections on the work in a new context yet to be significantly represented in the literature of the field. Debra Kalmanowitz and Bobby Lloyd's *Art Therapy and Political Violence* (2004) presented a similar global perspective by describing practice in settings that range from the Balkans to the Middle East, Sudan, Northern Ireland, New York, South Africa, and Sri Lanka, but this is the first study examining art therapy throughout Asia and documenting how the region assimilates approaches developed in other countries, creates its unique home-grown practices, and potentially influences the future international development of the discipline.

The authors make a major contribution to art therapy, not only in terms of international expansion, but to the exploration of comparative practices in different parts of the world. As I read the chapters in the book I found myself examining the whole of art therapy through an Asian lens as well as considering applications to the many regions in this vast territory.

Regarding issues of cultural influence, my primary reaction was in sync with the editors' – Kalmanowitz, Jordan Potash, and Siu Mei Chan – perception of productive tensions that permeate the overall discourse, presented poetically in the book's subtitle, *To the Bone or Wrapped in Silk?* We might ask: what aspects of art therapy embody and engage cultures, regions, and places; are there features that transcend these differences; and to what extent are universal and local qualities combined into a yin and yang of art therapy?

---

1   More than 60 per cent of the world population is in Asia, with approximately 37 per cent in China and India, as contrasted to 5 per cent in North America (US Census Bureau).

One of the greatest compliments I can give to *Art Therapy in Asia* is that it presents more questions and possibilities than answers and thus expands and sets the stage for future dialogue, research, creation, and professional development within a global context. The issues summarized by the editors in the beginning and concluding chapters apply to Asia and every other part of the world.

It is noteworthy to see how the collection of chapters describing Asian practice contains the broad spectrum of theoretical orientations that exist in North America, Western Europe, the Middle East, and Australia. In this respect there is a relative constancy to differences of practice rather than the hegemony of a singular paradigm. However, while presenting these variations the book will not disappoint readers hoping for a strong articulation of art therapy advances informed by Asian philosophical traditions, approaches to health, and contemplative practices.

Because of their relevance and appeal, these principles have been integrated into the worldwide practice of art therapy beginning with C.G. Jung's early 20th century practice of active imagination and continuing today in the writings of art therapists and training programmes like Naropa University in the United States. Seminal concepts and actions have a way of flying over boundaries of every kind and reaching people who are receptive to them via creative contagion. However, there is special relevance and authority when art therapists working within the regions of Asia apply principles and practices which are widely understood and naturally accepted by the people they serve. This is new and the most important contribution of *Art Therapy in Asia*, which can inform research in other places and, as the authors suggest, lead to more detailed studies within Asia.

Rather than trying to impose alien psychological notions, many chapters view creative expressions as manifestations of the vital energy, qi or chi, which Asians know so well. In keeping with the principles of Chinese medicine, art therapists concentrate on the activation and circulation of energy which finds its way to areas of need and provides the basis for a transformative process of artistic healing. I was intrigued to see art therapy adapted to tai chi in China and how people were receptive to the movement basis of painting and drawing.

Participants in art therapy familiar with Buddhist, Taoist, and yoga traditions were perhaps able to instinctively grasp the therapeutic significance of painting as a contemplative process and physical practice of aesthetic harmony that can have a corresponding impact of larger spheres of experience. The Buddhist concentration on the present moment, beginner's mind, sensations, constant change, compassion, the interconnection of all things, and sensitivity for the limits of spoken language and conceptualization arguably presents one of the most natural theories of art therapy practice in Asia and beyond. The same can be said of the book's description of the Indian aesthetic encouraging the interrelationship of all of the senses and artistic disciplines. And the whole of art therapy can benefit from the authors' embrace of Asian approaches to incremental transformation and change, and demonstrations of how art therapy can be integrated into daily health practices and the pervasive sense that each small action is part of a larger Karma of influences within the person and communities.

The Asian context also presents unique problems and challenges. How does one practise art therapy in communities where the expression of personal conflicts and negative feelings is traditionally viewed as threatening the larger social harmony?

How do art therapists trained in the North America, Europe, and Australia operate in Korea, China, and Japan where it is common to suppress personal emotions which are fundamental to the art therapy experience?

The authors show how potential difficulties present opportunities for expanding and adjusting the scope of art therapy. They embrace what comes innately to people such as the effects of aesthetic factors and the process of communicating with others through art. Cultural orientations to collective experience are used to affirm how a person is not isolated 'on an island' and is part of a larger and necessary web of interconnected people.

The way art therapists in Asia and the people they serve deal with these problems and find meaning through the process of art making holds great promise for art therapy everywhere.

Art Therapy in Asia embraces the complexity of cultures, human differences, and universal aspects of experience. For example, the authors ask whether the notion of being Asian is a composite of factors, in no way monolithic. They similarly avoid sweeping statements and stereotypic labels about differences between the relative notions of East and West – that is, the former being more holistic and the latter individualistic – and appreciate how variations within groups are often more significant than those between the designated types. The identification and affirmation of differences is an infinite process of human individuation known well to experienced therapists and thus we have to keep a careful eye on any effort to reduce people to cultural categories. In therapy we look closely at individual lives and problems and how they are influenced by culture, language, geography, nationality, religion, moral codes, family structures, socio-economics, politics, education, and the endless and unique variables of particular situations.

The chapters of this book give many examples of how art therapists engage these issues, and the editors suggest their personal take on the interplay of universal elements and cultural differences when they say, 'The art therapy sessions may follow familiar Western patterns, while the way in which the therapist chooses to relate to the child, adult or parents may contain all the cultural nuances necessary to communicate the importance of the therapy itself' (p.47).

As the practice of art therapy grows internationally together with the needs to advocate and communicate, I trust that the prevalence of English in art therapy literature and training will change. Language, English perhaps followed by German and Dutch, is the only current area of cultural dominance that I observe in the field, but the increasing translation of books into Japanese, Chinese, and Korean will stimulate an increase of writings in Asian languages as we currently see in French, Russian, Hebrew, Portuguese, and Spanish.

On the basis of my four decades of international involvement with art therapy and studies of world traditions of art and healing beginning with an examination of connections between art therapy and shamanism, a word with Northern and Central Asian origins (McNiff, 1979, 1984), I continuously ask, how are we different and the same? Interestingly enough the shamanic and indigenous healing traditions from throughout the world consistently define illness as a loss of soul and treatment as soul retrieval, an idea that applies beautifully to what we do today in art therapy, and especially to Asia if we substitute the word soul for the Chinese qi. I was intrigued with how perhaps the most classically Chinese of the chapters, 'Landscape of the Mind', is closely attuned to my making of artistic sanctuaries where imagination heals by furthering the circulation of creative energy in ways that sometimes bypass plans and expectations.

While this book advocates appreciation of contextual and regional variables, it also helps us see what art therapists everywhere have in common, and what the traditions of Asia contribute to the whole.

The empirical and basic things that we do in art therapy practice tend strongly toward the universal as confirmed throughout *Art Therapy in Asia*. All art therapists strive to create safety, support expression with art materials, guide the process, witness the expressions of participants, make assessments, and document outcomes within a more general attempt to establish a creative space that holds the overall work.

Although culture and many other variables influence the materials, contents, and styles of artistic expression and attitudes towards images that we see in art therapy practice, the fundamental actions and emotional effects of drawing, painting, sculpting, collage, photography, and the use of the wide spectrum of other media offer a basis for objective and cross-cultural study, all of which can be conducted before we begin to discuss symbols, theories, and psychological meanings which tend to multiply into a plethora of interpretations influenced by culture, beliefs, personal backgrounds, individual interests, perceptions, and the creative imagination.

Among the many things that an Asian perspective on art therapy offers is the need to give closer attention to the significance of artistic actions and attentive witnessing in the present moment. In every region of the world clinical practice can observe and assess how people move with materials; the rhythms and tempos of actions; degrees of relaxation and concentration; and abilities to deal with structural and graphic challenges, sustain participation, engage others, respond imaginatively, and describe personal reactions to artistic processes and the communications of images.

Physical experience can thus be viewed as the great common denominator in art therapy like the breath in contemplative practice. When verbal language and especially approaches based more on a particular psychology or ideology become primary in therapeutic practice, universality tends to be more limited – different languages further amplify cultural variations. The worldwide discipline of art therapy involves varying partnerships between these primary features.

No matter what theories are used to inform practice or languages used for discussion, the bodily and emotional qualities of working with people individually and in groups with art materials tend to be more similar than different across cultures. In addition to the observable actions involved in the making of objects, every form of art therapy generates relatively permanent forms of artistic expression that exist independently. And it is remarkable how children and beginning artists in all regions of the world show great similarities in working with basic media such as drawing, painting, collage, and clay. These commonalities of innate experimentation with materials contrast to the artistic traditions formed through training in particular methods, genre, and styles which can vary dramatically and create the misleading perception that primary forms of graphic expression differ significantly across cultures.

In my practice I consciously move toward elemental ways of engaging art materials in order to be more inclusive and lower obstacles to expression which tend to be attitudinal and common to people (McNiff, 2009). Simple methods as reinforced by Asian contemplative disciplines (Suzuki, 1989) also further artistic and psychological depth by focusing attention and offering relatively unbiased structures and stimulations for free expression.

The images presented in the chapters describing art therapy experiences in China, Korea, Hong Kong, Japan, the Philippines, Cambodia, Taiwan, Thailand, Singapore, and India in many ways closely resemble the range of art therapy expressions that I have seen in other regions of the world. For example, pictures made with colour markers are consistent in graphic and pictorial qualities. The same applies to moulding with clay and collage which is distinctly influenced by the colours, texture, and shapes of the things used to form a composition. The qualities of a particular medium have a major impact on what the hand, eye, and imagination are able to do with them.

As the authors note, improvisational gestures tend to generate artistic expressions that transcend cultural forms, especially when enhanced by unfamiliar and new media. Asia's traditions of spontaneous and minimal brush strokes, new to most people in other parts of the world, present art therapy with a time-tested basis for furthering natural expression. I find these gestures more artistically expansive than the prevailing art therapy practice of making linear scribbles. And yet paradoxically it is the most free-flowing of all painting media, brush work with ink, that engenders restraint in the example given in the chapter 'Reflecting on Materials and Process in Sichuan, China', underscoring how there are no absolutes in this discourse on art, therapy, and Asia. Familiar and ingrained cultural use of a particular medium which in this case elicited traditional subjects (bamboo, blossoms, and empty space) can trump imaginative experimentation.

As a researcher looking at how art heals I find that, once people are able to get past inhibitions, fears, and resistances, the process of art making has a transformative and healing effect which happens on the level of creative energy (qi) and emotion. The Sichuan art therapy participants confirm what I hear from people in other parts of the world who experience the curative effects of art making after dealing with obstacles to expression which may play a necessary role in activating emotions. The healing effects of art therapy have so much to do with opening, trying something different, engaging difficulties, building self-confidence, stabilizing emotions, relaxation, and a resulting sense of creative satisfaction that ensues from immersing ourselves in this process and trusting its intelligence.

The mainstream of art therapy practice, as demonstrated in this book and the recent literature in the field, is moving increasingly toward an appreciation of artistic processes and energies as primary medicines, ways of knowing, and vehicles of change. Objects are less likely to be reduced to concepts or split off into the process–product dualism that previously characterized the field. The artistic image is a necessary participant in the process of creation, an interconnected whole that involves action and reflection, people and objects, yin and yang. We do not have to go far from art to explain what we do as images, creative action, energies, relationships, challenges, difficulties, and communities of people are increasingly viewed as partners in creation and healing. These directions are very much in sync with the wisdom and traditions of Asia.

The dialectical and open-ended spirit of inquiry that permeates *Art Therapy in Asia* is refreshing and good medicine for art therapy. The book challenged me at every turn, making it necessary to look at the other side of my most familiar positions. The best things happen when people from throughout the world and from vastly different backgrounds listen to each other, study their respective traditions and ideas, open themselves to communion and influence, and move beyond ideologies of separation to mutual influence and creation.

Shaun McNiff, PhD, ATR, HLM, is the First University Professor at Lesley University in Cambridge, Massachusetts, USA. A past President and Honorary Life Member of the American Art Therapy Association, he is the author of many books, three of which have been translated and published in Chinese (*Art as Medicine; Art-Based Research*) and Japanese (*The Arts and Psychotherapy*).

References

Kalmanowitz, D. and Lloyd, B. (2004) *Art Therapy and Political Violence.* London and New York: Brunner-Routledge.

McNiff, S. (1979) 'From shamanism to art therapy.' *Art Psychotherapy 6*, 3, 155–161.

McNiff, S. (1984) 'Cross-cultural psychotherapy and art.' *Art Therapy: Journal of the American Art Therapy Association 1*, 3, 125–131. (Re-published 2009, 25th Anniversary issue of *Art Therapy: Journal of the American Art Therapy Association 26*, 3, 100–106).

McNiff, S. (2009) *Integrating the Arts in Therapy: History, Theory, and Practice.* Springfield, IL: Charles C. Thomas.

Suzuki, S. (1989) *Zen Mind: Beginner's Mind.* New York, NY: Weatherhill.

Foreword

William Fan

Everything should be made as simple as possible, but no simpler.

(attributed to Albert Einstein)

I travelled in the wilderness and met three gurus painstakingly catching fragments of paintings flying everywhere in the air. They were collecting as many of these fragments as they could and trying to re-image/re-imagine them into a holistic picture with all their wits. I admired their efforts but could not but wonder whether they could ever collect enough fragments to piece together a cohesive picture. Moreover they might come from more than one picture. My scepticism had to be explicit on my face, for the gurus smiled and handed me a few of these fragments glittering in the sun.

'These are pieces of Thang-ka,1 paintings believed to be endowed with power to facilitate meditation and enlightenment within our faith. We are sorting them into different categories to make easier the piecing together. We hope to understand, learn and benefit about the embedded meanings and energy.' They softly explained to me with eyes lit with aspiration.

I looked closely at the fragments and instantly became intrigued by the complexities and variations as well as uniqueness in each of these fragments. There were obviously common themes linking them together while there were equally contrasting features keeping them apart.

Then I realized that my doubts were of no avail. We should just appreciate each of these fragments on its own merit to benefit from the embedded power of enlightenment through our own meditation and self-reflection. They are not meant to be dissected from their context and

---

1   Thang-ka are Tibetan Buddhist paintings or embroidery for meditation and enlightenment, usually covered with silk.

analysed to the molecular level. The sorting might make things easier for the novice but the exploration would not stop there. Unanswered questions were often more thought provoking and inspiring than half-boiled answers. This had to be a personal journey.

So, I expressed to the gurus my appreciation of their kind efforts and thoughtful deeds and spent some happy times leisurely looking through the collected fragments in random order, to savour them each according to my own inclination. I even caught a few flying fragments with my own hands and read them before letting them blow away into the air. Magically I started to feel more relaxed and serene as I realized that these paintings were made to communicate and to interact with the readers.

I bowed in thanks to the three gurus and returned to my unfinished journey.

The above vision developed in my mind when I was pondering on how to fulfil the invitation of writing a foreword to this voluminous compilation which not only breaks virgin ground in Asia, but also stands at the forefront in the conceptualization of the many cultural issues in art therapy globally.

It is rather paradoxical when we consider that we are here concerned with art, a human activity/attitude/orientation, which is so readily put at the other end of the balance with science, that the editors have chosen to take up a very philosophical and thinking approach in editing this book. Readers will certainly agree with me that this book is a science book on art healing. The three editors have scholastically revealed their many considerations and decisions in the course of the editing and even reviewed their own limitations. Readers should take heed to read the first two and the last chapters written by the editors, even if they decide to thumb through the other chapters in a random manner as I personally prefer.

All philosophy as well as science may be regarded as a search for unity in the attempt to comprehend the diversity of things under general principles or laws. In analytical (convergent) thinking, there is always this issue of defining and differentiating concepts. This inevitably leads to the argument between the dichotomies, such as in art critique the persistent argument about content and form, in philosophy the physics and metaphysics, in psychology the body and mind, and in psychiatry the brain and mind. In intuitive (divergent) thinking, we are more concerned about gaining a holistic and wholesome impression or personal meaning.

Maybe even the notion of the West and Asian is but another of these dichotomies, and only serves to form the two arms of a scale. We can then strike a delicate balance by adding and extracting weights on the two arms to find out how art heals.

Judging from the subtitle *To the Bone or Wrapped in Silk* chosen for the book, the question most endearing to the editors' hearts/minds is: how much should the native Asian cultures be integrated into art therapy which has been formalized into a therapeutic entity in the West? This difficulty of course arises only because the editors have opened up the term 'art therapy' from the narrow sense of art psychotherapy to the wider sense of art healing. This recalls in me the lingering question of how Asians would adapt psychoanalysis into their cultures. While art is integral, spiritual, intuitive and beyond words by nature, art therapy can hardly be reduced to analysis or interpretation by the rational mind. Readers are open to cast their votes after reading through the book.

The editors deserve great applause for their hearts, thoughts and efforts; I am delighted to be among the first to applaud.

This book should be on the shelves of everyone interested in art and/or healing.

William FAN, MD, is a specialist in psychiatry in private practice who worked for many years at Castle Peak Hospital in Hong Kong where he coordinated the Art-in-Castle Peak Hospital Project to promote the use of arts with mentally ill clients. He is also an Adjunct Associate Professor of Counselling and Psychology at Shue Yan University and serves as an Honorary Consultant for the Hong Kong Association of Art Therapists.

Chapter 1

Introduction to Art Therapy in Asia

Debra Kalmanowitz, Jordan S. Potash and Siu Mei Chan

A book on the relationship between art, art therapy, creativity and healing in Asia must go beyond mere historical fact in order to explore the heart, spirit and essence of culture and tradition. Our goal in bringing together this book is to document and record the diverse ways that art therapy is practised throughout Asia, as well as to try to understand what the influences are that are motivating the thinking and practice. In so doing, we have looked for indications of regional trends, examples of specific cultures, and examples of individual practice.

This book is a first attempt to present art therapy in Asia. It is undoubtedly complex to portray art therapy in Asia in one single volume, and given the enormity of this task, we acknowledge that this book can only serve to introduce and invite the reader to seek further to understand more about Asia. In addition to rousing the interest for further exploration, we hope that readers in all parts of the world will read this book and be inspired to learn and re-examine their own art therapy practices in light of these examples.

In this chapter we attempt to make implicit values explicit; we also attempt to understand the culture-bound values that influence art therapy in Asia. Although many academics recognize that there is great variety within any culture, there are also certain trends and patterns that run across the diversity of cultures that exist within Asia. Often these larger patterns address such areas as the role of the individual within family and society, holistic conceptions of health, the place of creativity and art, religion and spirituality, all of which play a linking role. Other links come about from migrating populations, political relationships, and shared conditions, culture and art.

Defining Asia

We hear references to Asia in relation to current events, art traditions, religious practices and political governance, which gives the impression that there is a single Asian system. Given the diversity in geography and cultures, one has to wonder if there really is an Asian way. Asia is a vast region that incorporates all of the countries bordered by Japan in the east to India in the west and from Indonesia in the south to China in the north. This demarcation is sometimes referred to as 'Pacific Asia' (Borthwick, 2007) or 'Monsoon Asia' (Murphey, 2008). This area covers diverse climates and landscapes, as well as cultures, languages, religions and politics. Due to proximity, sometimes Australia and parts of the Middle East are considered Asia, although culturally they are quite different, even in the face of cultural diversity within Asia itself. If there is a distinct Asian culture, then it has its roots in Hinduism and Buddhism from India, Confucianism and Taoism from China, and many folk beliefs and ancestral traditions from individual countries and regions (Scupin, 2006).

The countries we are covering are each unique and it is not our intention to dull these differences. Despite the diversity and the different ways in which each country is modernizing and growing, there are many roots in common and enough patterns to follow. They represent a group which is becoming more and more interdependent, particularly since the Asian financial crisis of 1997, when many of these countries strengthened their regional alliances and developed some institutions specifically for Asia (Palmer Kaup, 2007). Indeed each country deserves a book on its own, and yet if we fail to look at the region as a whole, the picture we get will be decidedly narrow. It is our hope that, by pulling these together, a bigger picture will form, which in turn will inform each one specifically. Throughout this book, we will typically refer to individual countries and cultures, so as to avoid giving the impression of a pan-Asian value system. At the same time, just as individuals refer to Europe despite differences among the individual countries, we will at times refer to Asia when it makes sense to do so.

Why document art therapy in Asia?

Before going far into this book, we should pause and ask why it is important to document art therapy in Asia as separate from the growing body of global art therapy theory and practice. Many art and arts therapists have stressed the importance of understanding the dominant values and the unexamined influence of Western cultural norms on art therapy practice (Campbell *et al.*, 1999; Hiscox and Calisch, 1998; Hocoy, 2002; Lewis, 1997; McNiff, 1984; Moon, 2006; Talwar, Iyer and Doby-Copeland, 2004). Within the West, this dialogue has taken place primarily among those who work with socially and culturally diverse populations to assure that art therapy practice is relevant to all. To meet this goal, Talwar (2010) stated:

> I assert that art therapists need to situate research and scholarship related to identity and difference within larger historical and social contexts – beyond, in other words, the monolithic or unitary narrative of art therapy. (p.12)

She demonstrates how a false belief in a single way of theorizing and practising art therapy limits an embrace of the wide spectrum within art therapy, its accessibility to clients of all backgrounds and the future development of the field. In this regard, Hocoy (2002) specifically mentioned the areas of engagement, treatment goal setting, structure, ambiguity and interpretation as to how art therapy may be accepted or misunderstood by clients from different social and cultural backgrounds. As one strategy in ensuring cultural relevance, Talwar (2010) offered that art therapists should begin by taking an 'intersectional perspective', which she defines as 'locating individual differences within the specific social and cultural experiences of individuals, rather than within a linear, unifying theory' (p.16). By embracing this approach, we can learn what constitutes art therapy in Asia on its own, not limited to Western ideas and assumptions.

Even while documenting unique aspects of art therapy, we are also cognizant of similarities and cross-fertilization between cultures. The world is increasingly unified as a result of globalization. It is not only the world's economic order, but the world's technological, sociocultural and political factors, in part due to the cross-border circulation of ideas, language and popular culture. In such a world, where there is communication and exchange between most parts of the world, there is an increasing movement towards each other, learning from each other and an integration of ideas, philosophies and practice. There is no doubt that Asian ideas have become part of Western psychological practice; with a contemporary example being the explosion of interest in mindfulness, and the creation of Western psychological techniques incorporating this concept (Kabat-Zinn, 1994). Asia, too, is integrating lessons from the West; an example of this is the embracing of Western medicine for particular illnesses and conditions. Exchange is inevitable and is happening, and therefore understanding each other and ourselves becomes increasingly pertinent.

This book attempts to understand art therapy practices in Asia. Our search in this regard is to understand the theories and practices within the contexts in which they arise. We do not and cannot assume that what constitutes art therapy in Asia is the same as what constitutes art therapy in the West, but at the same time we do not want to assign an assumed difference based only on cultural and geographic difference. Through documenting and examining art therapy throughout Asia, we can come to see where culture influences, informs, interferes or explains. As the number of art therapists increases throughout Asia, as a result of growing opportunities for training and interest in gaining international experiences, there is a growing need to understand the values and practices that shape art therapy in Asia.

Review of art therapy in Asia

Part of our reason for writing this book relates to the relative lack of literature on art therapy throughout the region. There are documented accounts of Western art therapists who visited different countries in Asia and reported back on their observations of art therapy (Arrington, 2005; Case, 1990; Stoll, 2005). There are also some reports of art therapists based in Asia who provide descriptions of art therapy in their own countries (Kim, 2009; Park and Hong, 2010).

Besides history, development and present conditions that provide a context for art therapy in different countries in Asia, there are some descriptions of practice by both local and visiting art therapists. Several art therapists in Korea (e.g. Kim *et al.*, 2006) wrote on the use of computers to assist and improve upon interpretation of art-based assessments. Wegman and Lusebrink (2000) documented the limits of using Western scoring techniques for kinetic family drawings by children in Taiwan. Silver (2003, 2009) documented the use of the Silver Drawing Test as an assessment in Thailand, but did not indicate if the scales required adjustment to account for culture differences. Although not necessarily art therapy, Got and Cheng (2008) demonstrated how sustained art-making workshops in Hong Kong with Chinese adults with developmental disabilities showed improvements in social relationships and language comprehension. Golub (2005) described her work in a psychiatric centre in China with implications for how cultural and political differences may inform art therapy. Chilcote (2007) described her humanitarian work in Sri Lanka in response to the devastating tsunami.

There are also examples of art therapy practices that point to implications of art therapy in Asia, even if they occurred in other parts of the world. Davis' (2010) study of 19 international students studying in Australia included 17 students from Asia. She found that art therapy helped them to express themselves by translating experiences into images that they had difficulty expressing in words due to either language or low acceptance of Western-style psychotherapy and counselling practices. As an example of a Japanese practice, Warner (2001) described her coordination of a Japanese lantern floating ritual in the US to coincide with the Japanese *bon* festival to demonstrate solidarity in commemoration of the bombing of Hiroshima.

We know that this review is limited in large part due to access and language, as there are many locally published accounts of art therapy in individual art therapy association newsletters. While these reports constitute an important body of country literature, they are not accessible beyond members of their association. The examples listed here represent documentations of experience, but lack a critical analysis of underlying values and assumptions. It is this point, in particular, that we hope to address in this book.

Brief overview of the development of art therapy in Asia

Like other parts of the world, the uses of arts in healing and ritual are very much a part of the diverse cultures throughout Asia. From the intricately created Kalachakra mandala of Tibetan Buddhists to the detailed carvings of deities at Angkor Wat, images have been used to educate and inspire, while also serving as foci for storytelling and meditation. Although other art forms may be more prominent, such as dancing or singing, the visual arts are evident in folklore, costumes and decoration. As in the Western world when the rise of science and the industrialized age diminished 'superstitious' belief systems, in Asia, colonialization caused a degree of devaluing of traditional health practices in place of the more Western ones. With new belief systems coming into being, the ancient use of the arts in healing may have been altered or marginalized, but they were not lost.

More recently pioneer artists, nurses, mental health workers and teachers developed models of working within their specific work frames. They thoughtfully created art-based models in their settings through their practice inspiration and sensitivity. These individuals developed their methods of working mostly unaware of the existence of an art therapy discipline.

In addition to the indigenous pioneering use of the arts in healing, there has been much contact between Asia and the West over time. The primary contact that Asia had with the West was a result of curious and entrepreneurial explorers, and the economic benefits often mixed with political objectives and business encounters. Individuals on both sides have learned from each other. The interactions have promoted a rich communication and exchange of the way in which different ways of thinking can inform art therapy theory and practice.

The development of art therapy in Asia is as diverse as the countries themselves. Attempting to fully document it is well beyond the scope of this book. What is clear is that across the vast region, and even within individual countries, there are a mix of indigenous practitioners, locals inspired by foreigners and those who sought education abroad. Whether as a result of age-old practice or accidentally discovering the healing benefits of art for particular populations, individuals in every country found how offering art can help. Sometimes art is used as a recreational activity, sometimes for its soothing capabilities, and sometimes for its expressive potential. This history, although on the other side of the world, mirrors the development of art therapy in the West.

'To the Bone or Wrapped in Silk'

During early stages in the development of this book and in particular conversations about what types of chapters to include, our colleague Ivy Fung posed the question, 'Is the art therapy practice Chinese to the bone or is it just wrapped in silk?' Widening her concern beyond Chinese applications of art therapy, we can ask if Asian art therapy practices are fundamentally different from Western approaches or do they simply use different metaphors and symbols? What we discovered was that this distinction is not always clear given the many factors involved in art therapy including health approaches, types of materials, metaphors, and understanding of processes. Furthermore, sometimes the use of culturally relevant symbols or metaphors, even if offered in a Western way of working, can serve as a bridge between cultures and help to engage an individual.

In attempting to identify an Asian practice, we did wonder if we could identify a Western one. At first, the question seems absurd given the diverse ways that art therapists practise in the West. Gilroy and Skaife's (1997) experiences as British art therapists at the annual conference of the American Art Therapy Association illustrate just some of the differences within Western art therapy. There are the ongoing debates on the relative importance of art or therapy, the role of graphic diagnostic indicators of health, and those who stress the need to focus on individuals, families, communities or society. Yet, despite this disparity there are commonalities, based on the Western value system and shared art history that is fundamental to art therapy practice. Even though there are art therapists who work outside of or against the traditional medical model and established high art traditions, they operate in an environment that accepts culture-bound values, that is those values so engrained in daily living and working that they go unnoticed and are taken for granted (Sue and Sue, 2007). It is exactly this idea that can be applied to Asia.

We should remember that each of the chapters represents a particular perspective. They are not intended as representative and we should be careful to remind ourselves that no culture is monolithic, as even within one culture individuals can have different perspectives, practices and beliefs (Caughey, 2006). Where possible, we have tried to honour this point by purposefully selecting multiple voices from the same countries in order to avoid the implication that the authors were the sole ambassadors of their particular country or culture. For every way of working described in this book, there are other art therapists throughout Asia (and indeed the world) who work in both similar and opposing ways.

The chapters for this book were selected primarily from an open call for proposals. Although we were inspired by the presentations at the Asian Art Therapy Symposium in Hong Kong in March 2009 (and some of the papers presented there are included in this volume), we deliberately opened our search as wide as possible. We contacted art therapists who we knew were working in Asia and those we discovered through networking groups, publications or those who received the call for papers from others. We asked for contributions related to theories and practices, imported, integrated, adapted or indigenous, which can inform art therapy in Asia. We specifically did not include purely descriptive accounts of history and development, as we wanted to maintain a focus on theory and practice, while avoiding the inherent power dynamics involved in who is appointed to be the recorders of history at the expense of those stories that are left unwritten. As editors, we have been careful to ensure that the chapters remained authentic and true to the authors. We chose to represent a range of voices including indigenous practitioners, locals who trained abroad, expatriate residents and guest trainers. All of them to some degree have contributed to, and represent, the development of art therapy in Asia. At the same time, we know that there are missing voices. There are those we know who were either unable or unwilling to participate, those we met too late into the publication process, and those we do not know. We expect that this book will be a start of documenting art therapy in Asia and we look forward to subsequent editions and publications.

Structure of the book

This book is divided into six major sections according to themes that emerged from an analysis of the chapters. Chapter 2 introduces each of these themes and sets the context for understanding their implications to art therapy in Asia. Following this overview, the book unfolds with examples from each area.

'Part 1: Views of Health' shows how uniquely Asian conceptions of health can inform and guide art therapy. The first two chapters, one by Gong, and the other by Richardson, Gollub and Wang, describe approaches to art therapy that incorporate Traditional Chinese Medicine. What differentiates them is that the first describes a synthesis that begins in art therapy, whereas the second describes how art was added into traditional healing. In the last chapter in this section, Kim describes how art therapy can accommodate both art and medicine to provide treatment, prevention or improvement of symptoms through art making.

The next section, 'Part 2: Influence of Collectivism', provides examples of how collectivist values interact with art therapy. Essame provides an overview of collective values and shares guidelines for how they inform her art therapy practice in Singapore. Lee and Byrne respectively describe case examples of how collectivist ideas can inform work with families and the elderly.

Recognizing the role that spirituality plays throughout Asia, 'Part 3: Integration of Spirituality' provides examples of work, while underpinning the importance of paying attention to the spiritual dimension of working. Pluckpankhajee describes the attraction to anthroposophic art therapy given its similarities to Buddhist values, which are at the base of Thai culture. Chua also describes Buddhism as to how it informs both her general art therapy practice and her work specifically with Buddhist clients. Taking an approach that emphasizes Japanese sensibility to mindfulness and contemplation, Rappaport, Ikemi and Miyake make a case for art therapy and art making based in Focusing.

'Part 4: Role of Art Traditions' considers how specific art traditions, processes and history affect the use of art in art therapy. Liang describes the philosophical underpinnings of Chinese brush painting and how these ancient ideas inform her modern-day art making. Singh turns to the traditional Hindu and Ayurvedic teachings on the connection between the arts and health. Potash and Kalmanowitz re-examine Western assumptions on art materials and the art therapy process in the context of their work in Sichuan, China. Emphasizing how traditional symbols can provide a sense of identity, Herbert demonstrates how the Cambodian arts can heal socio-political upheaval.

While all of the sections provide strategies for working, 'Part 5: Models of Art Therapy,' offers practical guidelines for working throughout Asia. Sezaki explains the importance of finding the right level of structure for his work in Japan in order to allow for maximum therapeutic benefit. Lu offers an assessment she developed for her clients in Taiwan, but has implications in other countries. Seeking to introduce expressive art therapy to her Chinese clients, Chang provides Chinese metaphors that can inspire expression.

Art therapy in the context of natural and man-made tragedies and in the context of a more transient world are covered in 'Part 6: Looking at Contemporary Asia.' Alfonso and Byers show how their humanitarian work in the Philippines was provided in a culturally appropriate matter that promoted strengthening relationships. Tan addresses human trafficking and the role of art therapy in individual healing, relationship building, and political advocacy. In closing, Finney describes her personal journey to discover a community as she navigated the terrain between Thai values and her Western art therapy training with her re-integration into Thailand.

In the last chapter of the book, we provide a summary of the themes and their implications for what might constitute an Asian model of art therapy.

References

Arrington, D.B. (2005) 'Global art therapy training – now and before.' *The Arts in Psychotherapy 32*, 193–203.

Borthwick, M. (2007) *Pacific Century: The Emergence of Modern Pacific Asia*, 3rd edn. Boulder, CO: Westview.

Campbell, J., Liebmann, M., Brooks, F., Jones, J. and Ward, C. (eds) (1999) *Art Therapy, Race and Culture*. London: Jessica Kingsley Publishers.

Case, C. (1990) 'Collectivism and individualism, the "We" and the "I": Art therapy in Hong Kong.' *Inscape* (Summer), 2–9.

Caughey, J.L. (2006) *Negotiating Cultures and Identity: Life History Issues, Methods, and Readings*. Lincoln, NE: University of Nebraska Press.

Chilcote, R.L. (2007) 'Art therapy with child tsunami survivors in Sri Lanka.' *Art Therapy: Journal of the American Art Therapy Association 24*, 4, 156–162.

Davis, B. (2010) 'Hermeneutic methods in art therapy research with international students.' *The Arts in Psychotherapy 37*, 3, 179–189.

Gilroy, A. and Skaife, S. (1997) 'Taking the pulse of American art therapy: A report on the 27th annual conference of the American Art Therapy Association, 13–17 November 1996, Philadelphia.' *International Journal of Art Therapy 2*, 2, 57–64.

Golub, D. (2005) 'Social action art therapy.' *Art Therapy: Journal of the American Art Therapy Association 22*, 1, 17–23.

Got, I.L.S. and Cheng, S.-T. (2008) 'The effects of art facilitation on the social functioning of people with developmental disability.' *Art Therapy: Journal of the American Art Therapy Association 25*, 1, 32–37.

Hiscox, A.R. and Calisch, A.C. (eds) (1998) *Tapestry of Cultural Issues in Art Therapy*. London: Jessica Kingsley Publishers.

Hocoy, D. (2002) 'Cross-cultural issues in art therapy.' *Art Therapy: Journal of the American Art Therapy Association 19*, 4, 141–145.

Kabat-Zinn, J. (1994) *Wherever You Go, There You Are: Mindfulness Meditation*. New York, NY: Hyperion.

Kim, S. (2009) 'Art therapy development in Korea: The current climate.' *The Arts in Psychotherapy 36*, 1–4.

Kim, S., Ryu, H.-J., Hwang, J.-O. and Kim, M.S.-H. (2006) 'An expert system approach to art psychotherapy.' *The Arts in Psychotherapy 33*, 1, 59–75.

Lewis, P. (1997) 'Multiculturalism and globalism in the arts in psychotherapy.' *The Arts in Psychotherapy 24*, 2, 123–127.

McNiff, S. (1984) 'Cross-cultural psychotherapy and art.' *Art Therapy: Journal of the American Art Therapy Association 1*, 1, 125–131.

Moon, B.L. (2006) *Ethical Issues in Art Therapy*, 2nd edn. Springfield, IL: Charles C. Thomas.

Murphey, R. (2008) *A History of Asia*, 6th edn. New York, NY: Longman.

Palmer Kaup, K. (2007) *Understanding Contemporary Asia Pacific*. Boulder, CO: Lynne Rienner.

Park, K. and Hong, E. (2010) 'A study on the perception of art therapy among mental health professionals in Korea.' *The Arts in Psychotherapy 37*, 4, 335–339.

Scupin, R. (ed.) (2006) *People and Cultures of Asia*. Upper Saddle River, NJ: Pearson Prentice Hall.

Silver, R. (2003) 'Cultural differences and similarities in responses to the silver drawing test in the USA, Brazil, Russia, Estonia, Thailand, and Australia.' *Art Therapy: Journal of the American Art Therapy Association 20,* 1, 16–20.

Silver, R. (2009) 'Identifying children and adolescents with depression: Review of the stimulus drawing task and draw a story research.' *Art Therapy: Journal of the American Art Therapy Association 26,* 4, 174–180.

Stoll, B. (2005) 'Growing pains: The international development of art therapy.' *The Arts in Psychotherapy 32,* 171–191.

Sue, D.W. and Sue, D. (2007) *Counseling the Culturally Different: Theory and Practice,* 5th edn. New York, NY: John Wiley.

Talwar, S. (2010) 'An intersectional framework for race, class, gender, and sexuality in art therapy.' *Art Therapy: Journal of the American Art Therapy Association 27,* 1, 11–17.

Talwar, S., Iyer, J. and Doby-Copeland, C. (2004) 'The invisible veil: Changing paradigms in the art therapy profession.' *Art Therapy: Journal of the American Art Therapy Association 21,* 1, 44–48.

Warner, D.A. (2001) 'The lantern-floating ritual: Linking a community together.' *Art Therapy: Journal of the American Art Therapy Association 18,* 1, 14–19.

Wegman, P. and Lusebrink, V.B. (2000) 'Kinetic family drawing scoring method for cross-cultural studies.' *The Arts in Psychotherapy 27,* 3, 179–190.

Chapter 2

Critical Themes of Art Therapy in Asia

Debra Kalmanowitz, Jordan S. Potash and Siu Mei Chan

For the Chinese, Confucius is considered a sage. He was a man who was practical and charismatic. His life, teachings and philosophies emerged slowly, organically. He had students, who were considered men of wisdom and virtue. Each of these men was also seen as a seed, and each seed slowly, but surely, spread their wisdom far and wide (Yu Dan, 2010). This notion of natural and balanced growth can be found in China's Creation myth about Pan Gu who separated the heaven and the earth:

> Heaven and earth were jumbled together in a cosmic egg for eighteen thousand years, and Pan Gu lived in the midst of it. The heavens and the earth split apart. The pure Yang essence became the heavens, the heavy Yin essence was the earth. Pan Gu was between them, nine changes in one day, a god in the heavens and a sage on the earth. Every day the heavens rose higher by ten feet, the earth grew thicker by ten feet, and Pan Gu became ten feet taller. When he reached eighteen thousand years of age, the heavens were infinitely high, the earth was infinitely deep, and Pan Gu was infinitely tall. (Yu Dan, 2010, p.13)

This separation was not sudden, but was a slow, long and lengthy process, calm and gentle, but nevertheless powerful, just like the way in which the sea slowly erodes the rocks in its path, forming soft, round shapes. The way this split between the heavens and the earth is described explains to us that the *change* was gradual. A gradual separation of light, yang, which became the heavens and heavy essence called yin, which became the earth. It seems that in this myth the creation is important, but equally emphasized is the Chinese idea of change. When we read this story we see that Pan Gu grew slowly, and had 'nine changes in one day'. Change is not described in Chinese philosophy as a big bang, which creates everything at once, but a gradual process (Yu Dan, 2010).

The use of art in healing in Asia has developed in the same way. The marriage between art and therapy, art and healing, art and medicine and art and the psyche has grown slowly. A formation of what has always been known into an attempt to adapt it to a disciplined thinking suitable for our time and place, suitable to this region. It is not by chance that a creation myth is chosen to begin this chapter, as making art, the act of artistic creation, has the capacity to fulfil a 'fundamental human instinct for transcendence' (Eliade, 1992, p.xii). This transcendence by its very nature alludes to transformation and change and through this to the creation of a new form.

The grounding principle of balance and gradual change is fundamental to the Asian psyche. Today, with the modernization of many of the countries in the region, the pace of life has become quicker. Hong Kong, Thailand, Singapore, Taiwan and Japan are just some of the countries represented in this book which have modernized, and live lives that parallel Western values, yet are still underpinned by their very varied cultural heritages. Tortoises or turtles (Figure 2.1) are revered, and sometimes seen as sacred in many myths, and depicted across Asia as animals that are easygoing, patient and wise (Walters, 1993). They are also seen as slow and peaceful creatures that symbolize longevity and stability. Turtles are seen in Chinese culture, and in India, Taiwan, Japan and Vietnam, and although the details of the mythology may vary from country to country, the symbolism across these countries remains the same. The traditional value of slow, solid stability leads to longevity, prosperity, harmony, tenacity, power and good luck. The gradual change described in the myth is pervasive in all aspects of traditional life and thinking and also serves to describe the nature of the therapeutic practices that evolved in Asia. Traditional treatments for illness, for example, tend to involve a longer-term approach aimed at enhancing health and wellbeing, with the treatment of symptoms being secondary.

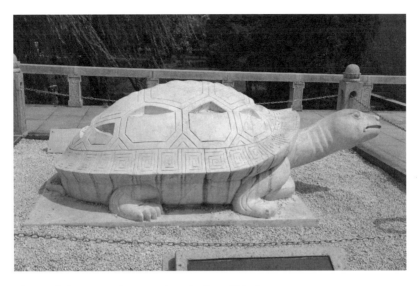

Figure 2.1 *Tortoise (Panmen Gate, Suzhou, China)*

Before looking at models specific to Asia and before we look at art therapy theories and practice that have emerged, or interventions that have been designed, we need to address those areas that point to the influences that may come into play when developing a unique Asian-based discipline and practice of art therapy.

Views of health

Ancient Greek civilization had a strong influence on the Western mind. The value placed on the logical-analytic system of thought of modern science can trace its roots to this civilization. Such an analytic style of thinking supports the detachment of an object from its context. The emphasis is placed rather on defining the object and categorizing it, creating rules by which to understand the world or the specific phenomenon. Different civilizations, such as Indian, African, Chinese and Native American, however, have recognized more holistic, more connected methods of knowing, of practice and philosophies (Lee *et al.*, 2009).

Health/illness and body/mind are seen as dichotomies in the West. Indeed, it is not only health/illness, body/mind and science/art that are separated. Today, we give great value to specializations. We define, focus and divide our knowledge, and practise creating specific, but often contrived, boundaries in the service of expertise, so much so that we have almost forgotten that everything is connected. Today we do not connect the body to the mind, although research (Cohen and Miller, 2001; Cohen *et al.*, 1998; Dalton *et al.*, 2002; Vitaliano *et al.*, 1998) has shown the strong connection between stress and cancer and susceptibility to immunity and respiratory infection, for example.

Kleinman (1980) perceived culture as part of medicine and not vice versa. For him the differentiation between illness and disease is important, because this gives us a clue as to how to treat patients and to an extent how to understand patients and their illness better: '*Disease* refers to a malfunctioning of biological and/or psychological process, while… *illness* refers to the psychosocial experience and meaning of perceived disease' (p.72). In other words, illness is influenced by culture, belief and society, and these beliefs and norms channel the illness experience and patient roles. In addition it is the way we think and make sense of things which indicates the relationships between patients and healers and illness and healing, and their cultural context. We can therefore say that there is a cultural construction of illness that can be looked at and extrapolated to other illnesses and other cultures.

Traditional medicine is part of a cultural heritage of every society, with most traditional models of medicine evolving as part of a culture. Despite the differences, many traditional systems have numerous aspects in common:

• The fundamental belief that there is no differentiation between body, mind and spirit and that health is a state of balance within the individual's body, as well as between the individual and the environment.

• Traditional medicine follows a holistic approach to diagnosis and treatment. It views the person as a totality, within a context, and will usually not only tend to the illness or symptoms, but to the system as a whole.

• Traditional medicine will suit the treatment according to the specifics of the individual within their specific context, and not apply the same medicine to different people even if the symptoms seem to be the same (World Health Organization, 2001).

The two main systems of traditional medicine in Asia are Traditional Chinese Medicine (TCM), native to China, and Ayurveda, traditional medicine, native to India. These traditional systems of medicine are highly developed and well documented. Both of these systems have impacted on many systems in neighbouring countries; TCM, for example, has impacted Japan, Korea, Vietnam, Taiwan and Thailand, which then developed their own variations. Ayurveda has impacted on countries in the region also, for example Thailand, Malaysia, Indonesia, Sri Lanka, Tibet and Burma. In addition to these two great traditions, the region also contains a number of simpler traditional practices, which are often passed down orally and have been developed between small and isolated ethnic groups (World Health Organization, 2001).

Topley (1970, 1981) traced the history of TCM from a spiritual and sacrificial system in the Chou dynasty (1122–934 bc) to the incorporation of ideas on equilibrium as observed in nature and finally to the integration of charms and amulets from Taoism in the T'ang dynasty (ad 618–906). The origins of healing as being associated with religion, divination, sacrificial offerings and later Buddhism, Taoism, Zen and Confucianism are common to many of the countries in Asia. The human body is seen as a microcosm of the universe, which is ruled by the complementary qualities of *yin* and *yang*, as well as phenomena whose basic characteristics are determined by the balance, excess or deficiency of *qi* (energy) according to the Five Elements (Figure 2.2) (O'Brien and Xue, 2003). The medical theory of equilibrium and balance is, according to Topley (1970, 1981), a single aspect of a more general theory of equilibrium and balance that is put forward to explain the nature of all phenomena, including society. Human beings are seen as a microcosm of the universe, a notion that extends to other phenomena in our universe too. This means that there is a connectedness between man and nature and interconnectedness between all things.

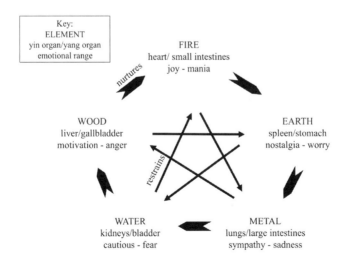

Figure 2.2 *Five Elements in Traditional Chinese Medicine*

Balance is fundamental to the Ayurvedic tradition too, and is emphasized in its philosophy and belief that lack of balance will lead to illness. Several philosophers in India combine religion and traditional medicine. The philosopher Nagarjuna is known chiefly for his doctrine *Mādhyamaka* (middle path); he wrote the medical works *The Hundred Prescriptions* and *The Precious Collection*, among others. Ayurveda, like TCM, is a holistic health system, which fosters the natural harmony between body, mind and soul. Ayurveda considers the human being as an inseparable unity of body, mind and soul. Instead of dealing only with the health or disease of separate organs, the wellbeing of the whole person is emphasized (Pole, 2006).

The foundation of scholarly medicine in Asia today is often less religious than metaphysical. Many of the countries in Asia are socially heterogeneous and are rapidly changing, making the subject of *traditional* versus *modern* medicine very important. Many Asian countries practise Western medicine, and the younger generation know, and perhaps care, very little about traditional methods of healing and ritual. There is no doubt, however, that traditional notions carry through, even if only through superstitious ideas (with their origins unknown). It is this way across the globe. No matter where we come from, we are influenced by ideas, thoughts and traditions, many of which we have no conscious knowledge. Within this complex subject, Eastern traditions point to holistic health by reminding us that separation is contrived and that all aspects of life influence each other. As art therapists, this attitude is compatible, as art therapy by its very nature is a combination of disciplines, bringing together the arts, the psyche, healing and health.

Influence of collectivism

In Asia, it is commonly believed that a person is not an individual living on an island, but is seen in context as a product and integral part of family, society and environment. Nisbett (2003) pointed out that, in a very general way, Asians tend to see themselves as interdependent and strongly identified with their group identities. This de-emphasis on individuality goes as far as the lack of a single word for either *I* or *individual* in many Asian languages. Instead people often refer to themselves by identifying their roles in relation to another (e.g. referring to oneself as a parent, alumni or nickname depending on the context).

Meta-review research on the extent of differences in individualism and collectivism between Asians and Westerners reveal a more nuanced picture than conventional wisdom tends to yield (Oyserman, Coon and Kemmelmeier, 2002). While Westerners tend to be more individualistically oriented compared to Asians, they are not necessarily less collective. Still, the importance of collectivism for Asians – as a stated value – is one that is well ingrained.

In trying to tease out how expectations of individualism have permeated Western psychological ideas, Lam (1997) postulated that, whereas Western ideas of adolescent development are focused around autonomy and individuation, a Chinese conception

> involves a process of developing, of connecting and of relating. The ultimate goal is to develop a web of good-fitted, harmonious, appropriate, socially accepted and additive interpersonal relationship networks in the adult world. The criteria for maturation, therefore, becomes: whether or not an adolescent is appropriately positioned in his/her social network and to what extent an adolescent is capable of mastering both vertical and horizontal interpersonal relationships. A concept of 'self-in-relational network', in contrast to an 'autonomous self', is therefore a better description of the unique experiences and developmental processes of Chinese adolescents. (Lam, 1997, p.108)

To understand how this difference affects health practices in TCM, for example, Maciocia (2009) explains that the concept of an individual self as an autonomous psychological being influenced and formed by intricate and multiple past experiences does not exist in a Confucian philosophy, and by extension in Chinese medicine. He considers the example of anger as seen through the eyes of Chinese medicine. Anger makes *qi* (energy) rise, and the correct treatment therefore consists of making qi descend. It does not investigate deeper into the person's psyche as to whether the anger may have its roots in past relationships, for example, or whether it may be due to childhood experiences. Chinese medicine does not seek psychological insights because such insights require a concept of an inner life and an autonomous individual self that Chinese culture does not have.

Although today in our post-modern world art therapy takes its influences from many cultures and philosophies across the globe, its origins as a Western discipline come from a Western individualist outlook. Art therapy as a Western practice is still guided by individualistic ideas such as self-expression, individual rights, and the art object as a personal statement (Case and Dalley, 1992).

Integration of spirituality

A discussion of the treatment of mental and emotional problems should look at the concept of the mind and spirit in Chinese medicine. The *Little Oxford Dictionary* (1986, as cited in Maciocia, 2009) definition of 'spirit' highlights an important feature of this concept in Western philosophy and illustrates its difference from Chinese philosophy. The dictionary's opening definition of 'spirit' is 'The animating or vital principle' (p.535) in humans which gives life to the physical organism.

This definition 'illustrates the duality between body and spirit that has been typical of most Western philosophy, a duality that is absent in Chinese medicine' (Maciocia, 2009, p.1). Chinese medicine conceives the 'spirit' as a refined form of matter. The 'spirit' includes all mental phenomena (thinking and reason, including that of the Ethereal Soul), emotional phenomena and bodily phenomena. This term is used without any reference to a particular religion and no inference is made on the spirit's destiny after death. According to Chinese medicine, the unity of spirit and body is central. The spirit is not something that brings the body alive. Instead, spirit and body are but two different states of qi. Both spirit and body are manifestations of qi, the spirit being the most rarefied form (Maciocia, 2009). The above distinction is significant as this means that there is no distinction between physical and mental health – all are just health.

Although Maciocia is addressing Chinese medicine specifically, the absence of dichotomy is true in Asia as a whole. In Ayurveda it is recognized that the human being is essentially a spiritual being and that the more we suppress our spiritual expression, the greater the attrition to health (Pole, 2006). Thai medicine, for example, traces its history back to a rich cultural heritage, from its origins in Buddhism, animism, Ayurveda, Kmer mysticism, TCM theories and indigenous beliefs in spirits and ghosts, to the formation of the healing tradition practised in both rural and urban Thailand today (Salguero, 2007).

As previously mentioned, two distinctive characteristics of Eastern philosophies are the centrality of balance and the inclusion of spirituality in the view of health. Reality is perceived as constantly changing, growing and developing, and within this moving world our challenge is to maintain balance. Spirituality is brought into treatment or therapy

> primarily through the recognition of the inseparability between human beings and nature (as postulated by yin–yang perspective and Daoism) and a transcendence of the self so

that one can shift the focus from the 'small self' to the 'big self' (as suggested by Buddhism). (Lee *et al.*, 2009, p.26)

The Buddhist teaching of the 'middle way' advocates for living less in the extremes and more in balance. There is a de-emphasis on excess feelings and emotions or on any behaviour that would upset individual and social harmony. The Taoist depiction of the yin–yang emphasizes both balance and interconnection. One of the lessons of this symbol is that there is no way to remove one aspect of life, as its opposite is dependent on it and in many ways a reflection of it. It should be mentioned that spirituality should not be confused with religion, but rather as a more general concept related to how people perceive their connection with others and the universe (Nhat Hanh, 1976).

Role of art in society

The various Asian cultures all have made significant and interesting contributions to the art world. Traditional Asian art includes the individuality of each separate nation, culture and ethnic group, but also possesses a collective similarity in design, style and traditional content. Influences across Asia spread and germinated between cultures. In addition an overlap of Buddhism, Confucianism and Taoism led to the adaptation of ideas from one Asian country to another. The art of Asia, especially China and India, was influenced by religion and philosophy. Confucianism, Hinduism and Buddhism – and later Christianity and Islam – played a part in the art of these lands, while at the same time these cultures influenced others in Asia. The influence of China on Korea, for example, is seen in the techniques borrowed from the Chinese who introduced their style of writing to Korea during the Bronze Age, while the mandala, which was meaningful in Japanese art as a representative of the universe and universal principles, is a symbol which comes from early Buddhist art (Hesseman, Dunn and Saptodewo, 1998).

When considering the role of art in Asia we are again obliged to go back in history. The religions of the world have always reacted to, and shaped, the world of images, and Asia is no different. Some of the teachers of China, for example, seem to have a similar view on the value of art as Pope Gregory the Great. They considered the importance of art as a means of reminding people of the great examples of virtue from the past (Gombrich, 1995). The most important motivator, however, came to the Eastern art through the influence of Buddhism. Buddhism influenced art in this region, not only by suggesting subject matter, but introduced an entirely new approach to images, to art in general. The religion of the East taught that 'nothing was more important than the right kind of meditation' (p.150). Meditation according to this Eastern philosophy means to ponder, or think about one thing for many hours, 'to fix an idea in one's mind and to look at it from all sides without letting go of it' (p.150). This according to Gombrich is an exercise which is common in Asia, and considered more important than physical exercise. The connection to the subsequent style of art that developed in Asia is expanded upon by Gombrich:

> That is, perhaps, how religious art in China came to be employed less for telling the legends of the Buddha and the Chinese teachers, less of the teaching of a particular doctrine – as Christian art was to be employed in the Middle Ages – than as an aid to the practice of meditation. Devout artists began to paint water and mountains in a spirit of reverence, not in order to teach any particular lesson, nor merely as decorations, but to provide material for deep thought. (Gombrich, 1995, p.150)

The intersection of art with the principles of health as a balance has resulted in part in an aesthetic that emphasizes harmony. Until recently, throughout Asia it is common to find images with subject matter related to religion, nature, festival observance and daily living. The intersection of harmony also influences subject matter that focuses on an individual's relation to nature, or to the gods. In terms of formal elements, compositions often appear balanced. In addition to the subject matter, the technique is often just as important as the imagery. This is evident in the age-old techniques of calligraphy and Chinese paintings, where the individual is encouraged to paint as if like a meditation. Here the traditional painting may be seen as an aid to meditation, an opportunity to ponder on life and provide material for deep thinking (Gombrich, 1995). We return to this in Chapter 14, Reflecting on Materials and Process in Sichuan, China (Kalmanowitz and Potash).

The earliest civilizations used art for healing, ritual, expression and communication (Dissanayake, 2007). This observation is true across cultures despite the fact that styles may be different, origins of content may vary and the fluctuation of society in allowing freedom or limitations of expression may shift and change. Art continues to play an integral and controversial role in society. In Indonesia, for example, artistic creativity is seen as an aid to building a bridge between the living and the inhabitants of the other world, whether they be deities, ancestors or spirits. It is often not very important who created the work of art; the artist remains in the background. What is important is *why* an object was made, and its function. Presumably it was not until after the encounter with the West that artistic objects were made not only for religious use but also commercial use (Hesseman *et al.* 1998).

Jumping forward to today, contemporary art has changed throughout the region, just as it has in the rest of the world, although the historical, traditional origins still seem to reverberate throughout Asia. Contemporary art today resembles each other both in the East and the West, taking influence from each other, and learning from each other, by defining both similarities and also by defining differences. According to Adorno (1997), a German sociologist, philosopher and musicologist, who writes on the critical role of art in society, art has a 'truth content' (p.29). In our contemporary world, Adorno maintains that art allows for the expression of difference. He describes how art creates a degree of 'imagined freedom' (p.30). This freedom is, however, not what we imagine; according to Adorno (as cited in Bolanos, 2007), this freedom makes us sensitive to the discrepancies in which we live and, instead of providing answers, allows us to recognize that which is lacking. Adorno believes that, in the contemporary world, art can represent the contradictions of society, and can participate in the dialogue as a culture counter to the accepted culture or ideology. This way of viewing the role of art is quite a leap from the traditional one we just represented, and somehow, somewhere, they live together.

In addition to the religious and community aspects of art, contemporary artists throughout Asia can provoke awareness and perhaps voice opinions that society may not address. In China, Ai Wei Wei has become a well-known artist and political activist who, by combining a very personal expression with his traditional Chinese heritage, manages to provide a contemporary narrative and uses his art to comment on politics in China. In India, Devi Prasad, a potter, painter and photographer, also combined his art with political activism. He was also a lifelong pacifist and peace activist and he promoted the ideals of Mahatma Gandhi. Rather than view them as separate worlds or professions, Devi tried to harmonize his politics and his art into an ethical and conscionable whole.

Models of art therapy

Throughout the world, there are many models of art therapy. Each model takes on a different psychological theory and comes from a different philosophical orientation. Art therapy can take its orientation from psychotherapy, behaviouralism and cognitive and transpersonal approaches, as well as from medicine, education and community arts, to name a few. In this same way, the models continue to develop and grow in Asia.

Art therapy is in some ways influenced by specific models of therapy that have been in existence in Asia. Unlike Western mental health practices that primarily make use of talking and medication, health practices in Asia have often made use of a variety of interventions. Hwang and Chang (2009) describe how contemporary psychological treatment models in Japan and China draw from Buddhism, Taoism and Confucianism by making use of rest, occupational activity and mindfulness to assist clients living with a range of mental health disorders – Morita Therapy, for example. Ayurveda treatments include what are considered activities that can lead to healing, for example, meditation, mantra, pranayama and yoga asanas, in addition to herbal remedies for treatment (Pole, 2006). Girindraseknar Bose, the father of Indian psychoanalysis who developed theories independent of Freud even though they were contemporaries, emphasized the integration of exercise with talk therapy and dream interpretation (Akhtar and Tummala-Nara, 2005). TCM makes use of herbs and soups often in combination with various types of massage and movement. Using prescriptive activities may fall within Chen and Emory's (1998) observations of models of psychology in Taiwan that make use of structured and authoritative approaches to mirror expected hierarchical social order and treatments intended to benefit not only the individual, but the client's full social context.

The scope of practices often includes some aspects of the arts. Ink brush painting is seen as a meditative activity that can induce a calm mood both in doing it and in viewing the final product. In addition to the visual arts, the bodily movement of qigong and the chime of the bell serve as additional arts-based healing activities. An important distinction between these practices and contemporary models of Western art therapy, however, is that the described arts practices typically follow an expected routine with an overall health goal that is not limited to personal expression and meaning. Furthermore, all of these activities are not limited to the ill, but are seen as important daily practices to maintain health and wellbeing. Given the traditional use of the arts in service of self-cultivation, relaxation and meditation, it's not surprising that the field of art therapy has made tremendous gains in Asia.

In addition to specific theoretical orientations and models, particular practices of art therapy are influenced by practitioners' understanding of their cultural heritage. As we will see later on in this volume, the model of art therapy that develops in this region can look as different as the variety of models that exist in the West. Some individual art therapists may embrace traditional values, including them either overtly or covertly within their work practice, while others may follow a model which may not have traces of Asian sensibilities. This is not to say that the therapists themselves have not adapted their way of thinking, but it may be expressed through different ways. The art therapy sessions may follow familiar Western patterns, while the way in which the therapist chooses to relate to the child, adult or parents may contain all the cultural nuances necessary to communicate the importance of the therapy itself.

Contemporary trends in Asia

The countries we are covering in this book are amongst the most widely varied in the world. Despite their diversity, they also represent a group of countries that are becoming increasingly interdependent. Particularly since the Asian financial crisis of 1997, many of these countries have strengthened their regional alliances and developed some institutions specifically for Asia such as the Association of Southeast Asian Nations (ASEAN) and ASEAN Plus Three, designed to increase ties among the ASEAN states of China, Japan and South Korea (Palmer Kaup, 2007).

Policy makers and scholars have observed the growing influence of the region and responded in different ways. Some have taken this as an opportunity to interact and develop relationships, and some have established think tanks, while there has also been lobbying to counter the region's economic, political and social rise (Palmer Kaup, 2007). Interactions and relationships have developed not only for political gains, but also out of need and urgency. Natural disasters or political strife can cause a draining of existing services and resources, to which the West or other countries respond. In the process of helping, values and ideas are shared, creating a rising awareness and new hybrid models of working.

It is true that all of the above examples have great significance in the internal working and life of creating a contemporary Asian model for art therapy. Globalization and modernization mean that most of the countries represented in this book simultaneously hold on to their existing modernized world and a strong sense of pride in thousands of years of history. Gaining a background in cultural and historical traditions does therefore seem essential in understanding the region today. The issues that face Asia in general and each country specifically include economic, political, agricultural and environmental challenges within changing and shifting societies and values. The influence of globalization means that the traditional ideas and values exist within a contemporary context and world. Among the other struggles associated with governance and maintaining citizen wellbeing, politicians, educators, entrepreneurs and practitioners in Asia often need to negotiate the lines between adhering to, adapting or relinquishing cultural values in the face of contemporary needs.

Conclusion

At the beginning of this chapter we told the story of Pan Gu, who separated the heaven and the earth, emphasizing the notion of natural and balanced growth as a founding principle of the Asian psyche. We have shown that this same idea of balance and holistic thinking is echoed in health practices. Indeed, according to the Vedas (the ancient literature on Sanskrit), *Ayur* means life and *Veda* means knowledge. Ayurveda therefore is the knowledge of life and not the knowledge of medicine. According to Ayurvedic mythology, knowledge of life neither has a beginning nor an end (Pole, 2006), again pointing to the notion of a holistic being and a holistic attitude towards life, healing and health.

While this review cannot explore each country specifically, there is enough interconnectedness to explain art therapy in Asia and provide sometimes stark contrasts to the unmentioned and sometimes unrealized Western values embedded in art therapy theory, discourse and practice. The various authors serve as guides to the trends occurring in art therapy in Asia. By discovering connections among the diverse and developing approaches, we can gain a broader view of the region and what motivates and influences the varied ways of working and thinking. In so doing, we hope not only to get a picture of one of the world's most exciting regions, but also to provide clues as to how art therapy can continue to develop in other parts of the world.

References

Adorno, T. (1997) *Aesthetic Theory* [R. Hullot-Kentor, Trans]. London: Athlone Press.

Akhtar, S. and Tummala-Nara, P. (2005) 'Psychoanalysis in India.' In: S. Akhtar (ed.) *Freud along the Ganges: Psychoanalytic Reflections on the People and Culture of India* (pp.3–25). New York, NY: Other Press.

Bolanos, P.A. (2007) 'The critical role of art: Adorno between utopia and dystopia.' *Kritke 1*, 1, 25–31.

Case, C. and Dalley, T. (1992) *The Handbook of Art Therapy*. London and New York: Routledge.

Chen, S.H. and Emory, R.E. (1998) 'Clinical Psychology in Asia: A Taiwanese Perspective.' In: A. Bellack and M. Hersen (eds) *Comprehensive Clinical Psychology, Volume 10: Sociocultural and Individual Differences* (pp.343–348). New York, NY: Elsevier Science.

Cohen, S. and Miller, G.E. (2001) 'Stress, Immunity, and Susceptibility to Upper Respiratory Infections.' In: R. Ader, D. Felten and N. Cohen (eds) *Psychoneuroimmunology*, 3rd edn (pp.499–509). New York, NY: Academic Press.

Cohen, S., Frank, E., Doyl, W.J., Skoner, D.P., Rabin, B.S. and Gwaltney, J.M. Jr (1998) 'Type of stressors that increase susceptibility to the common cold in healthy adults.' *Health Psychology 17*, 3, 214–233.

Dalton, S.O., Boesen, E.H., Ross, L., Schapiro, I.R. and Johansen, C. (2002) 'Mind and cancer: Do psychological factors cause cancer?' *European Journal of Cancer 38*, 10, 1313–1323.

Dissanayake, E. (2007) 'What Art Is and What Art Does: An Overview of Contemporary Evolutionary Hypotheses.' In: C. Martindale, P. Locher and V.M. Petrov (eds) *Evolutionary and Neurocognitive Approaches to Aesthetics, Creativity and the Arts* (pp.1–14). Amityville, NY: Baywood Publishing Company.

Eliade, M. (1992) *Symbolism, the Sacred and the Arts*. New York, NY: Continuum.

Gombrich, E.H. (1995) *The Story of Art*, 16th edn. London: Phaidon.

Hesseman, S., Dunn, M. and Saptodewo, S.K. (1998) *The Art of East Asia*. Cologne, Germany: Konemann.

Hwang, K.-K. and Chang, J. (2009) 'Self-cultivation: Culturally sensitive psychotherapies in Confucian societies.' *The Counseling Psychologist 37*, 7, 1010–1032.

Kleinman, A. (1980) *Patients and Healers in the Context of Culture: An Exploration of the Borderland between Anthropology, Medicine, and Psychiatry (Comparative Studies of Health Systems and Medical Care, No 3)*. Berkley, CA: University of California Press.

Lam, C.M. (1997) 'A cultural perspective on the study of Chinese adolescent development.' *Child and Adolescent Social Work Journal 14*, 2, 95–113.

Lee, M.Y., Ng, S., Leung, P.P.Y. and Chan, C.L.W. (eds) (2009) *Integrative Body–Mind–Spirit Social Work: An Empirically Based Approach to Assessment and Treatment*. Oxford: Oxford University Press.

Maciocia, G. (2009) *The Psyche in Chinese Medicine: Treatment of Emotional and Mental Disharmonies with Acupuncture and Chinese Herbs*. London and New York: Churchill Livingstone.

Nhat Hanh, T. (1976) *The Miracle of Mindfulness*. Boston, MA: Beacon Press.

Nisbett, R. (2003) *The Geography of Thought: How Asians and Westerners Think Differently… and Why*. New York, NY: Free Press.

O'Brien, K.A. and Xue, C.C. (2003) 'The Theoretical Framework of Chinese Medicine.' In: P.-C. Leung, C.C. Xue and Y.-C. Cheng (eds) *A Comprehensive Guide to Chinese Medicine* (pp.47–84). Singapore: World Scientific Publishing.

Oyserman, D., Coon, H.M. and Kemmelmeier, M. (2002) 'Rethinking individualism and collectivism: Evaluation of theoretical assumptions and meta-analyses.' *Psychological Bulletin 128*, 1, 3–72.

Palmer Kaup, K. (2007) *Understanding Contemporary Asia Pacific*. Boulder, CO: Lynne Rienner.

Pole, S. (2006) *Ayurvedic Medicine: The Principles of Traditional Practice*. Philadelphia, PA: Churchill Livingstone Elsevier.

Salguero, C.P. (2007) *Traditional Thai Medicine: Buddhism, Animism, Ayurveda*. Prescott, AZ: Hohm Press.

Topley, M. (1970) 'Chinese traditional ideas and the treatment of disease: Two examples from Hong Kong.' *Man 5*, 3, 421–437.

Topley, M. (1981) 'Patients and healers in the context of culture: An exploration of the borderland between anthropology, medicine, and psychiatry.' *Journal of Asian Studies 40*, 2, 332–334.

Vitaliano, P.P., Scanland, J.M., Ochs, H.D., Syrjala, K., Siegler, I.C. and Snyder, E.A. (1998) 'Psychological stress moderates the relationship of cancer history with natural killer cell activity.' *Annals of Behavioural Medicine 20*, 3, 199–208.

Walters, D. (1993) *Chinese Mythology: An Encyclopedia of Myth and Legend (World Mythology)*. London: Aquarian.

World Health Organization (2001) *Traditional Medicine*. Regional committee, 52nd session (August 6), Brunei: Regional Office for the Western Pacific.

Yu Dan (2010) *Confucius from the Heart: Ancient Wisdom for Today's World*. London: Pan Books/Macmillan Publishers.

PART 1

Views on Health

Chapter 3

Yi Shu

An Integration of Chinese Medicine and the Creative Arts

Gong Shu

For centuries the processes involved in Chinese painting have been considered a spiritual exercise, a means for nurturing and cultivating *xin* (心, mind/heart). Xin is translated as mind/heart, but also as mind and heart individually, thus demonstrating a unity of mind and body. Although in Western medicine the brain controls the whole body, Traditional Chinese Medicine (TCM) adheres to the heart as the master among the five yin and six yang organs that regulate the human body. As an example, "concentrate" in Chinese is 用心, which literally translates as using the heart, whereas in English it usually denotes putting your mind on something.

Nurturing the xin helps an individual break through the mental or emotional blockage that inhibits the natural process. In essence, Chinese painting can be construed as a form of mindfulness meditation. This practice is especially true of landscape painting where the artist meditates upon the spontaneous growth process of nature. The process initiates what Gestalt theory refers to as an "awareness continuum," a meditative state which focuses the senses and stops mind chatter by focusing on the here and now (Perls, Hefferline and Goodman, 1951). Research confirms that mindfulness meditation can produce psychological wellbeing and ameliorate many disorders, making this practice a powerful form of healing (Hölzel *et al.*, 2011).

How would one integrate the Chinese painting process into the practice of therapy or healing? What is therapy in general and what is art therapy in particular? For more than 30 years I have devoted myself to the study of healing and therapy. Throughout these years, I undertook training in psycho-imagination, guided imageries, radix, bioenergetics, psychodrama, and lastly TCM.

In the spring of 1977, when I was teaching Chinese painting, a student of mine told me that, ever since she studied Chinese painting with me, her insomnia of 20 years was cured. She asked me if I had ever heard of art therapy. In the fall of that year I enrolled in the art therapy program at Lindenwood College (now University) and received my master's degree in art therapy two years later. In the meantime I took Gestalt training. My master's thesis, "Awareness and Growth in an Art Therapy Practice," integrated Chinese philosophy and the theory of Gestalt therapy. It adopted the theory from the *Yi Jing* (*Book of Changes*), which states that the cosmos is an organic and unified whole. It emphasizes that the human body is not only unified within itself, but it is also inseparably unified with the natural world. The individual, the social institutions, and the natural world constitute an organic unity.

In the fall of 1993, I returned to Taiwan to participate in the 3rd Pacific Rim Regional Congress of the International Association of Group Psychotherapy. Since then I have been doing expressive arts training work in Taiwan, Malaysia, Singapore, and Mainland China. It was in October of that year that I was first introduced to TCM by a student at the Beijing Medical University.

My art therapy process also adopts the theory of spontaneity and creativity in Daoism which holds that every organism has an innate potential and tendency to sustain, enhance, and actualize itself. An organism will of its own accord function to find relationships of needs, potentials, and resources as long as its natural processes are not blocked. If they are blocked, growth is impeded. My work in Asia continues to help me integrate the healing processes of the East and West in the development of the therapeutic process that I call *Yi Shu*.

Tenets of Traditional Chinese Medicine

In TCM there is no such thing as psychotherapy. Due to its holistic perspective TCM treats the whole person and does not differentiate psyche from soma. It considers an individual an integral entity and an inseparable part of society, the natural world and the entire cosmos. The foundational philosophy and theory is from the *Yi Jing* (*Book of Changes*), which maintains that the world consists of five basic elements: water, wood, metal, fire, and earth. The theory of the five elements is used to explain the functions and processes of natural phenomena and of the human body with its five *yin* and six *yang* internal organs. The articulation of these internal organs corresponds to the diurnal and seasonal revolutions of the natural world. The changes in the phenomenal world outside affect individuals' internal processes: their psyche, soma, spirit, and *qi* (energy). More than 3000 years ago the Chinese understood the seasonal affective disorder.

TCM views human health from the perspective of *yin* and *yang* dialogical transformations. The visible, substantial, and tangible physical body is considered as *yang* in nature; whereas the invisible, insubstantial, and intangible energy body is construed as *yin* in nature. The *yin* and the *yang* elements co-exist at all times. They influence and transform into each other. Neither can exist without the other. In the healing process, when the energy body is healed then the physical body is healed as well. Conversely, if the energy body is off balance, the physical body will also suffer.

TCM considers illness a sign of *qi* energy imbalance in the body, which may be caused by environmental conditions or by human emotions. The external causes include changes of weather, wind, temperature, or levels of pollutants in the environment, or a person's unhealthy interaction with others or with the environment such as an unhealthy lifestyle. The internal causes of blockage and disharmony are usually a person's emotions. Emotional imbalance not only causes disharmony and imbalance in the body's internal organs, but it also impedes an individual's interaction with the environment. Health can be restored by changing one's lifestyle, by regulating the functions of the internal organs, by activating and harmonizing the *qi* in the body, and by harmonizing one's emotions.

Healing is a constant process of balancing the *yin/yang* energies in the human system and of bringing the individual to a natural state. Practices such as acupuncture and *qi gong* exercises are used to correct energy imbalance. Chinese landscape painting is also used to bring persons to what Perls *et al.* (1951) refer to as a "spontaneous sensing of what arises in you of what you are doing, feeling, planning" (p.75). The trouble is that traumatic experiences, which reside deep in the individual's body, mind, and spirit, causing the energy blockage, are not easily detected or healed.

The role of creativity and art therapy in healing

What is then the difference between art therapy and artistic creation? What distinguishes art therapy from artistic creation is that an artist will filter art works through virtuosity, a learned way of using artistic technique in the service of artistic vision. The forms they seek are shaped by their long training or self-discipline and their images of completion. Thus the work of art may not be a true or totally spontaneous embodiment of the actual feelings they are projecting. It may not contain all the raw materials of the original feelings and intuitions.

In an art therapy process, artistic quality and knowledge of the media are not the client's main concern. They are encouraged to express the uncontrolled "eruption of primary-process mechanism," because it is precisely the image of the clients' inner life not screened by the cultural context by which the work is judged (Arieti, 1976, pp.210–214).

There is of course a distinction between the experience of the client and the role of the art therapist in this creative process. The focus of therapy is on enhancing the client's awareness and personal growth, rather than on the aesthetic quality. The art therapist's role in this process is that of a facilitator and supporter. The therapist initiates and guides the client to fully concentrate on the creative process. For the therapist this too is a creative experience, calling on the therapist's own spontaneity as a resource to facilitate the client's process.

Let us look now more fully at the client's experiences of this creative process. I am using the word "implicit" to refer to psychic contents prior to their becoming explicit in the creative therapy process. For these contents, the decisive step of explicit creation has not yet been taken. They lack organization, or they are diffuse, indefinite, and unclear. Their changes occur without being clearly recognized. John Livingston Lowes (1927) spoke of "the surging chaos of the unexpressed" (p.13). The "chaos" is dynamic, constantly changing, full of tension and unrealized tendencies. The individuals are in a state where they cannot yet apprehend clearly what is there: what they feel, what is buried beneath the reach of awareness. This formless state is described by the poet Stephen Spender (1955) as "a dim cloud of ideas which must be condensed into a shower of words" (p.53). Langer (1967) speaks of this process in the following:

> The only adequate symbolic projection of our insights into feeling (including the feeling of rational thought, which the discursive record or rational order has to omit) is artistic expression… [The elements of a work of art] are all created appearances which reflect the patterns of our organic and emotional tensions so ostensibly that people are not ever aware of speaking figuratively when they speak of "space tension,"

"harmonic tensions," the "tension" between two dance partners, even between two works of art. Like a metaphor, it is to be understood without translation or comparison of ideas; it exhibits its forms, and the import is immediately perceived in it. (pp.103–104)

The contents, then, of implicit awareness are lived or expressed in creative work, in some medium, in an experience. Because art expression is in itself intuitive, involving the whole experiential perceptual process, it provides an easy and quick path for the client to come through these stages and acknowledge the previously unrecognized, blocked contents. The created image reveals much of the psychic reality of the creator.

As with the artist, so with the client undergoing art therapy. The client is in a state of vagueness, unclear about emotion, motive, and unfinished business, which have been suppressed, and repressed by the rules or regulations, the "shoulds" and "should nots" of the cultural conserve. This is where creativity begins. The mind is ready to disgorge the contents from which it suffers, to release this pressure and yield to the inward necessity of the individual, to what John Livingston Lowes (1927) calls the "hovering cloud of shadowy presence" (p.14). These unfinished situations are brought into the client's awareness through the creative process. It is here that the feelings are felt and expressed. It is here, in the art forms, that they are made manifest and explicit (Gong, 2004).

Yi Shu

Philosophy

From my studies in art, art therapy, Gestalt theory, and TCM, I have developed a treatment modality called *Yi Shu*. *Yi* means "change," *Shu* means "the way," the "art," or "the dao." *Yi Shu* simply means "the art of living with change." The fundamental thesis in *Yi Shu* is that healing is a constant process of balancing and harmonizing the psychological, biological, social, and spiritual realms of the self. *Yi Shu* embraces a wide range of therapeutic methods and forms of creative expression from both Eastern and Western cultures.

Philosophically *Yi Shu* follows the belief system of the holistic perspective, and the spontaneity and creativity of Daoism. It is process-oriented and its consciousness of space and time is dynamic and non-linear. It considers that the cosmic organism is in perpetual movement, a constant flow towards the union of the *yin* and *yang* opposites, towards harmony and balance. The cosmic energy that propels this movement is called *qi*. The *qi* that circulates around the natural world is the same *qi* that circulates in the human body. Besides *qi*, there is water that moves about the natural world. The blood and body fluid that circulate in the human body are analogous to the function of water in the natural world.

The major theories in the holistic perspective of TCM are the theory of *yin* and *yang* and the theory of the five elements. These elements precede one another during the cyclic evolution. They function to generate and restrict one another. The generating and restricting nature of the five elements are essential influences on the therapeutic procedures of *Yi Shu* in dealing with human emotions and their related energy imbalance in the body.

Spontaneity is the key to an individual's growth and development; all spontaneous body movements and behaviors are an individual's creative adjustment towards wholeness. Neurotic behaviors are seen as lack of spontaneity and are often characterized by *qi* blockage and *qi* imbalance or disharmony in a certain part of the organism. The blockage and imbalance can occur within the individual organism or in the individual's interaction with the environment. They keep an individual from participating fully in the moment of being.

According to the Daoist philosophy the natural and spontaneous innocence of a newborn baby embodies the state of truth, beauty, goodness, balance, and harmony. This state of spontaneity is called *zhen jin* or pure experience. This pure experience is analogous to the Gestalt awareness continuum. A person who achieves this state is called a *zhen ren* or an authentic person. To the Chan Buddhist and the Daoist, *zi-ran*, naturalness and spontaneity, is a way of achieving wholeness. *Zi-ran* simply means following one's nature and letting be, being spontaneous and not striving, being oneself, being fully aware.

Yi Shu attempts to demonstrate the uses of the creative process to achieve harmony and balance as in the authentic person. The authentic person verifies the theory of Organism as a Whole. It aims at helping individuals or groups to break through the impediment of energy blocks to reach harmony and balance in their relationships with themselves and with the world. The ultimate goal of *Yi Shu* is, then, to create a harmonious world.

Emotions are viewed as the invisible energy body, whereas behaviors and physical symptoms can be considered as the visible physical body. Emotional imbalance often affects the physical body. In the treatment of psychological difficulties *Yi Shu* treats not only the emotions or the energy body, but also the behavior, or the physical body. Through creative processes of art, music, dance, and drama, one makes the invisible visible and the intangible tangible; in these ways the emotional states are made observable. *Yi Shu* treats the tangible physical body and the intangible energy body simultaneously.

Implications for trauma

Traumatic experience buried deep in the psyche can best be externalized and concretized via various expressive arts including music, painting, dance, or dramatic enactments (Gantt and Tinnin, 2009). In addition to these creative arts, *Yi Shu* also employs the process of TCM in balancing and harmonizing the *qi* within and about an individual. The processes of *Yi Shu* can be used in individual sessions as well as in groups.

We know that full awareness is the key to creativity and growth. Blocks to awareness cause various conflicts in body, mind, and spirit and impede growth. There are many ways that awareness can be blocked. Awareness is blocked when individuals fixate their energy in the past, the future, and in conceptions or ideas that do not relate to the here and now. When this happens their innate urges and needs are neglected. These neglected and unattended needs and tendencies are what may be called the content of one's implicit awareness. They are called implicit in one's awareness because they are screened from one's full awareness. They are repressed or suppressed at the time of the original experience and thereafter denied to memory, or are regressed from original explicit states to a non-explicit level. This is true especially in the case of traumatic experiences.

Traumatic repressed feelings become chaotic but remain implicit in awareness until they are attended to and experienced. The forgotten images of traumatic experiences bind up one's energy and cause physical discomfort, such as a lump in the chest, a pain in the stomach, a headache, diarrhea, or constipation. The creative process of art therapy brings what is implicit and chaotic into an explicit state of being. Although the creative process of painting or doing art is in itself a therapeutic process, the images concretized in art therapy can be further explored in dramatic enactment and energy work adopting the process and theory of TCM and *Yi Shu*. In addition to these creative arts, *Yi Shu* also employs the process of TCM in balancing and harmonizing the *qi* within and about an individual. The processes of *Yi Shu* can be used in individual sessions as well as in groups.

Procedure

Let us now examine the procedures involved in the healing process of *Yi Shu*. The procedures begin with a meditative *qi gong*, a breathing and imaging process that aims at activating the two major meridians. The *dumai* meridian runs from the tip of the spine upward along the spine to the top of the head, and forward and downward through the face. The *renmai* meridian runs from the upper lip descending through the center of the chest, downward passing through the lower abdomen, to the tip of the spine, and allows the energy to go through the entire body and return to the earth through the center of the feet.

During the breathing and imaging process, I also guide the participants to visualize the colors that emanate from the universe, caressing and nourishing each corresponding internal organ in their body. The second step is to facilitate breathing and free body movements with music while imagining being surrounded by the colors of a rainbow. The music guides the group to take a journey of their souls into the deep unconscious. This process will help the participants become aware and open up energy blockages.

Following this exercise the participants are introduced to a painting process using Chinese painting brushes and papers. Traditionally as mentioned earlier, Chinese painting has been used as a spiritual exercise to foster spontaneity and creativity. It enables a person to externalize the inner processes experienced in the prior exercise. The Chinese painting brush and paper are chosen because of their yielding sensitivity. They register even a minute tremor of the hand. A drop of water on the paper will leave its mark forever. The process implicitly teaches us that life is like a Chinese brush stroke; once it makes its mark, it cannot be erased. One can only go on from here; there is no way to erase the mark or back-track. The painting registers the psychological gestalt of the painter. Figure 3.1 shows the paintings of a *Yi Shu* group in China in March 2011.

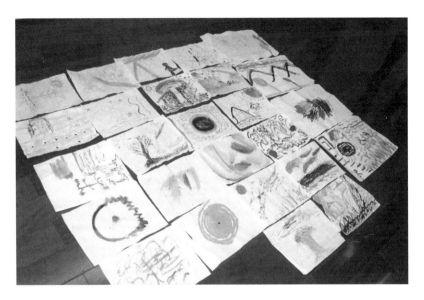

Figure 3.1 *Yi Shu group paintings*

The next step is to choose a painting from the group. Each of the images and colors, as well as the patterns of the color relationship in the painting, are enacted through movement or sound or both. The enactment externalizes for the individual the unconscious inner reality. The music, dance, and body-movement enable clients to have access to the hidden needs, urges, and innate inclinations that oftentimes are blocked from their conscious awareness. Painting externalizes for them the images of these inner necessities. As we notice from the above-mentioned procedures of *Yi Shu*, painting is the most important link in the healing process. It functions as a map that guides the client towards healing.

Case study: Judy

The following is a case study illustrating the procedures of *Yi Shu* and how art therapy functions in the process. This is the case of Judy, a 20-year-old Asian woman. She was referred to my group by her primary therapist. Although the group met only twice yearly for five days each time, the therapists working with the clients had intense supervision throughout the year. Judy participated in all the procedures of *Yi Shu*. She sat in a corner curled up in a fetal position for most of the first five-day workshop. During the second group session five months later, Judy was encouraged to come to the dramatic stage with her painting. Her painting showed a small figure lying in the middle surrounded by layers and layers of dark colors (Figure 3.2). She stood in a corner pulling her hair, hitting herself on the head, and refused to make eye contact with me. She growled like an animal and we had to protect her by restraining her. I encouraged her to lie down on a mattress as shown in her painting. She became terrified, mute, and shaking. She dissociated. I suspected that something must have happened while she was lying down. I asked her what had happened. She said in an inaudible voice "Daddy." When she was seven years old, her father came to her room and raped her.

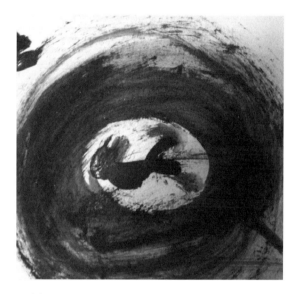

Figure 3.2 *Judy's painting*

I dimmed the light in the theater and had the scene re-enacted at her specification. A female auxiliary was chosen to play the perpetrator. This time she was able to pull the perpetrator away from the seven-year-old double and throw him off the stage. After the scene, I had her choose someone to hold her. Her therapist was chosen to comfort her. She rested her body on her therapist, heart to heart, while soft lullaby music was playing in the background. When she calmed down I had her dialogue with the seven-year-old and reassured the child that it was not her fault and that she was as pure as ever. Then I had her lying on her stomach and opened her *dumai* meridian and had her vomit out all the negative emotions and sounds she had swallowed over the years.

Dramatic enactment and TCM energy work channeled through *Yi Shu* helped her express her repressed feelings of anger, shame, and sorrow followed by love and nurturance from the group. I encouraged her to create an art journal to express her feelings every day and continue to work with her therapist. A year later, she began menstruating regularly for the first time, her breasts began to grow, her feet grew two sizes larger, and she grew two centimeters taller. She was able to hug and socialize with members of the group, as she had not been able to do with people for most of her growing years.

Painting helped her to express the traumatic feelings, which she was unable to express in words. The traumatic incident caused sudden unexpected fright in her and shocked her entire system, body, mind, and spirit, and it caused the energy to scatter and dissipate. In other words, the shock was so severe that it caused her entire system to shut down. The therapeutic experience altered her perception of the world from an environment of hostility to a place of love and compassion.

Art therapy was the major element in Judy's growth and healing. Her art journal continuously served as a guide for her work with her therapist. *Yi Shu* uses the process of creativity to bring to explicit awareness what is implicitly surging in one's awareness. In this process the therapist can help a client to release energy blocks for creative growth.

Conclusion

Just as Daoism believes that spontaneity and creativity are the core of healing and growth, so *Yi Shu* uses therapeutic procedures to enhance these processes to create a social environment that is conducive to creative growth. In order to create a healthy world, each and every one of us is responsible for remembering the integrity and beauty of each person and our own cultural heritage. We need to be open and free to welcome and appreciate the differences and the validity of the cultures of others without being enslaved by our own cultural perspective. By combining ideas from the East and West, art therapy functions as a major link in my therapeutic practice of *Yi Shu*. It serves as a map that helps individuals and groups bring out their inner conflicts and energy blockages that inhibit growth and creativity. It reminds us that, even in our current fast-paced world, we are all creators, not reactors or robots. So, let us work together to create a harmonious world.

References

Arieti, S. (1976) *Creativity: The Magic Synthesis*. New York, NY: Basic Books.

Gantt, L. and Tinnin, L.W. (2009) "Support for a neurobiological view of trauma with implications for art therapy." *The Arts in Psychotherapy 36*, 3, 148–153.

Gong, S. (2004) *Yi Shu: The Art of Living with Change. Integrating Traditional Chinese Medicine, Psychodrama and the Creative Arts*. St. Louis, MO: F.E. Robbins and Sons.

Hölzel, B.K., Carmody, J., Vangel, M., Congleton, C. *et al.* (2011) "Mindfulness practice leads to increases in regional brain gray matter density." *Psychiatry Research: Neuroimaging 191*, 1, 36–43.

Langer, S. (1967) *Feeling and Form*. New York, NY: Charles Scribner and Sons.

Lowes, J.L. (1927) *The Road to Xanado: A Study in the Ways of the Imagination*. Boston, MA: Houghton Mifflin.

Perls, F., Hefferline, R. and Goodman, P. (1951) *Gestalt Therapy*. New York, NY: Dell.

Spender, S. (1955) *The Making of a Poem*. New York, NY: W.W. Norton and Co.

Chapter 4

Inkdance

Body, Mind and Chinese Medicine as Sources for Art Therapy

Jane Ferris Richardson, Andrea Gollub and Wang Chunhong

We are writing this chapter in three voices. They are woven together in harmony with many different threads. Our collaboration in Beijing at the Third "Art and Natural Health Conference" in 2009 deepened our shared awareness of the role of both body and mind in the creation of art, and of new possibilities for art therapy practice. Wang Chunhong's concern as our host was to help her colleagues integrate Western art therapy approaches with creative Chinese approaches to healing. From the conference she realized the need for the cultures of East and West to work together to build art therapy theory and practice in China. The Western-trained art therapists also gained a new perspective, one that will be less familiar to some readers.

Wang, who is trained as a dancer and choreographer, is also trained in the Traditional Chinese Medicine theory of ZangXiang. She integrates her experience in healing, dance, and art into her own therapeutic approach that she calls DaDance Therapy. Wang feels that she must use all the dimensions of the arts (she includes Chinese medicine as an art) to heal all dimensions of the client's problem.

Art therapy in Beijing is in the beginning stages. Future art therapists from Beijing must study abroad, since the only university creative arts therapy program is in Music Therapy. Programs in Music Therapy are offered in eight different universities (Wang, 2009). Dimensionalartdance courses are also offered in many universities, thanks in part to the efforts of Wang. Dance therapy training is now offered in classified courses at Beijing Geely University. Wang created an International Conference to explore these interconnections between the arts and healing at a time of creative exploration and foundational development of art therapy in China.

Art therapy influences corresponding to DaDance therapy

Andrea Gollub and Jane Richardson's education at Lesley University took place near the beginning of art therapy master's level training in the United States. This training included a more eclectic and non-traditional therapeutic approach, one that is not always considered mainstream in the profession of art therapy. Our core professor, Shaun McNiff (2009), wrote about the connections between the expressive arts therapies and systems of healing based on a theory of correspondences, such as Traditional Chinese Medicine. This articulation was still to come when we began our graduate work. There was one published work that foreshadowed the integration of all the arts in art therapy, Florence Cane's (1951/1983) *The Artist in Each of Us*, with an emphasis on "free rhythmic use of the body in breathing, movement and sound" (p.37) as the necessary elements of painting. McNiff's work with his clients and students similarly drew on expressive movement as a source to inspire expressive art. This integration of the arts in therapy was similar to what we experienced in China.

Cane's daughter, Katherine Cane Detri (1983), reflected on this multimodal perspective in her foreword to the reprint of her mother's book. She discussed the training in various movement and relaxation techniques her mother received and then commented that her mother

> was open to every new wave of energy that helped free the human soul and body. She became involved with the new art of the 20s…later she became deeply interested in Eastern Philosophy. (p.iiii)

Cane explored the mind–body connection, and together with her sister, Margaret Naumburg, developed the scribble technique, which incorporated movement and breath awareness in the creation of a piece of artwork. Cane's deep familiarity with Jungian approaches made her very aware that the images which emerged could be coming from the unconscious of the artist, and could be used to help heal on a deeply integrative level. When we met Wang Chunhong, and witnessed her work, she struck us as akin to a Chinese Florence Cane. Our reading in art therapy history, our training with McNiff, and our experience of

Chinese traditional healing as acupuncture patients all helped to prepare us for our collaboration at the conference. In Beijing, we learned from art, and intuitively learned from one another.

The heart–mind and the heart print

The foreign therapists experienced both ancient and contemporary Chinese art as an integral part of the conference. We visited the Forbidden City and the 798 Dashanzi Art Center, where we saw contemporary paintings created with the traditional Chinese materials of brush and ink. We noticed that the ancient concept of heart–mind, or "hsin" (Sze, 1992, p.618), as a unified concept still seemed very present in much of the contemporary work. We learned that painting is traditionally discussed in terms closely connected to Chinese philosophy, and that painting actually shows us, through a visual language, the Chinese philosophy of life (Van Briessen, 1998), and beliefs about the heart, mind, and spirit.

Fu (2009), a presenter at the conference, described traditional Chinese healing as "an art of medicine" (p.42), that works, as art does, with the mind and spirit as well as the body. The traditional five elements of Traditional Chinese Medicine—wood, fire, earth, metal, and water—are as connected to art as they are to healing. The flow of energy is a vital process within the body, within art, and within the relationship of the artist and the painted world. This dynamic is equally true whether the artist is a young woman with special needs painting in therapy or an accomplished professional painter.

The Mustard Seed Garden Manual of Painting (Sze, 1992), a traditional text for the education of artists, discusses the concept of heart–mind as particularly significant for the painter. However, the heart and the mind are equally connected for the artist and the viewer within the traditional Chinese view of art, where "the act of painting is not separate from the flow of life itself, and painting is seen as infused with qi, or energy" (Richardson and Demaine, in press). This movement of qi is the basis of the first principle of Chinese painting, which is "Resonance of the spirit: Movement of life" (Van Briessen, 1998, p.110). When the connection between the inner spirit and energy of the artist and the outer form of the painting becomes visible, a painting may then truly be seen as a "heart print" (Hearn, 2008, p.106) of the artist, authentic and resonant. Yet the heart print is not an expression of emotion alone. As contemporary ink painter Qiu Ting (in Sheng, 2011) wrote of his painting process,

"I felt my hand and brush, heart and mind were all in the best possible partnership with one another" (p.172).

The traditional Chinese artist also works towards creating, "not so much a realistic imitation of the world around him, but rather… the expression of a mood or feeling" (Van Briessen in Richardson and Demaine, in press). The relationship implicit in a painting is always an important element of every artist's working process: a practice very congruent with that of art therapy, and also with Wang's DaDance therapy.

Wang weaves together art and movement in a seamless flow as she helps clients to integrate the heart and mind, and to develop the client's connection to the world. As a traditional healer as well as a creative arts therapist, she works within the framework of Traditional Chinese Medicine. The core concepts consist of balancing energy and working with the five elements, which are present in all living things. We Western therapists realized that she possesses an innate understanding of the "creative cycle" of the five elemental energies, which, together with the "control cycle," works dynamically in the balance and transformation of energy (Reid, 1994, p.52). In the Chinese view, the transformative process of art making is paralleled by the transformative movement of energy within the body.

The connection between the concepts of art and healing has been increasingly acknowledged in Western views of how art therapy works. As McNiff (2004) reminds us, "There was a time not long ago that the mention of the word healing evoked suspicion within the art therapy community." Now, as McNiff notes, "In the first sentence the present mission statement of the American Art Therapy Association declares that the making of art is, 'healing and life enhancing'" (p.3). In China, the power of art is, and has been for millennia, integrated into the system of healing. In Wang's practice, the application of Traditional Chinese Medicine to the practice of, and interpretation of, art therapy is seamless. The concepts of interpretation and diagnosis occur within a more holistic perspective than is commonly used in the West.

The five elements and art therapy

The theory of the five elements is important to the understanding of creative arts therapy practice in China. The five elements helped the Western therapists to understand how our Chinese colleagues worked with color, line, and movement in art making in therapy; and the five elements gave us an understanding of how they used diagnosis and interpretation in a holistic fashion to help their patients integrate their own energy and self-understanding. While all of the Chinese therapists understood these interrelationships, the Western therapists did not. In Wang's workshops, we experienced and felt connections between movement and mark making, color, and emotion. Reid (1994) describes these interrelationships, or correspondences, in the following way:

> The five elemental energies and their cycles provide a practical working model through which the interrelationships between the human body and the natural environment may be understood and controlled… All aspects of human health including physiology and pathology, diagnosis and therapy, are rooted in this remarkably reliable system of polar forces and cyclic energy transformations. (Reid, 1994, p.53)

Not only are the five elements connected with the organs and the flow of qi, or energy, within the body, but they are connected to both the language and practice of art therapy and the creative arts therapies through their correspondences with line, color, sound, and even taste. For example: The wood element which is Zang–liver and Fu–gallbladder is connected to the color–blue; the tone–Jiao 3; the moral–peace; the spirit–creative; the mood/mind–angry; the movement–control; the spread–slow; direction–up; and the taste–sour.

The five elements theory and the concept of yin and yang are simplifications of the "ZangXiang Theory" of Traditional Chinese Medicine. It is this more complex theory that helps Wang Chunhong decide when to use different elements like dance movement and art. ZangXiang helps her not only see the relationship between the organs, consciousness, and behavior, but also sound, color, movement, etc. Knowledge of these inner relationships helps Wang Chunhong decide whether she needs to work from the element of color to movement, or music to color, etc.

Painting the inner and outer worlds: example of Wang's DaDance therapy

We want to share an example of how Wang joins the heart and mind as she utilizes both movement and ink painting. A discussion of her use of these modalities in individual treatment provides a clinical context for her work. In this example of DaDance therapy, the increasing balance between the inner world of felt experience and growing awareness of communication with the outer world through creating art can be clearly recognized. Wang's young adult client, referred to here as ShiJing, had significant medical, emotional, and cognitive challenges. These included epilepsy and obesity, together with constant fevers of no known origin, with a bloated body, and an IQ of 42. Yet when ShiJing painted, she brought out a very special power, the power to express what she sees in her inner world. She used ink and color to express both what she sees with her eyes, and feels in her inner world, things she was unable to express any other way. It was easier to connect with and share this young artist's inner world by exploring her artwork with her.

Through DaDance therapy, ShiJing gained the ability to use the mediums of ink and color for expression of her experiences of both the outer scene and her inner world. Her IQ went up 56 points over her two years of treatment, and she began to have normal dialogues with ordinary people. She shed much of her fear of communication, and her fear of criticism. She gained the ability to express both what she sees and her personal connection to what is depicted in her paintings. She began to listen to others more openly, and to reflect on her own work and experience.

After five months of work in DaDance therapy, which included music, movement, Traditional Chinese Medicine, and ink painting, she created *Composing* (Figure 4.1). This painting represents an epiphany she had after doing a specific singing and movement exercise designed to help encourage movement of qi in the spleen or Pi (a water and valley element).

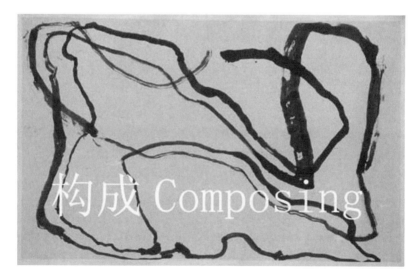

Figure 4.1 *Composing*

According to Traditional Chinese Medicine, Pi, which is different from the Western spleen, tells us where energy is needed in the body and what is required to balance it. The spleen controls the muscles. Dance helps to balance the energy of the spleen by increasing awareness of the body's nutritional needs and sending nutrition to the brain to help resolve issues of chaotic thinking. After she sang and danced, ShiJing said, "There is a brand new feeling, like all new and very large in my mind; these things are very clear." When asked "Like what?" she replied, "It is the constructing of a solid and stable new building, it's not done, but only a framework; the house is still vacant inside." She was then asked to draw Figure 4.1 using ink. Ink was used at first with ShiJing because ink helps make clients think more clearly and helps to organize the information from the movement and music exercises.

Wang frequently uses art to help solidify the process opened up by music and movement. In this case, art was used to solidify the scattered information in her mind. It was also a way to store the results of the session and strengthen the client's sense of positive growth.

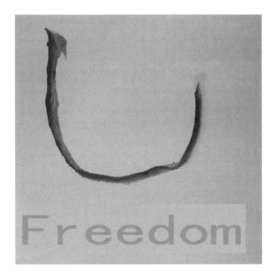

Figure 4.2 *Freedom*

The second elegant brush painting (Figure 4.2) further depicts the emotional and physical changes in this client. After eight months, ShiJing automatically used art to record her feelings after a session of music and dance therapy. She explained that the feeling in this picture was "freedom." When asked why, she asked, "What does it look like?" Wang replied, "A hook." ShiJing's response then was to ask, "Are there fish on the hooks? Fish do not bite, so they are free."

Since this exchange, her confusion has lessened significantly. She resolved the problem of her body and is now able to move more freely and make clearer choices. She is no longer impeded by and overly influenced by external factors. This change means that her heart is now strong and clear enough that she knows what she wants and can go after it, without fear. Ink and color were used throughout the eight-month phase of treatment, as treatment is not a straight line but a three-dimensional state, including body, mind, and spirit. However, after "Freedom," ShiJing was encouraged to use color more frequently because color can be used to help to understand development and mobilize courage. She has become very interested in art. Part of the therapy involves going on field trips to art galleries to see paintings and discussing the relation between color, structures, and materials. Now, ShiJing is able to understand the painting, and she is able to feel the artist's mood and what the artist wanted to express. Through this artistic appreciation she has been able to consolidate her own sense of purpose.

This young woman's striking paintings were viewed when the venue of the conference moved to the Beijing Olympic Mental Hospital, where she had an exhibition. She clearly had found the freedom to "go after" her self-expression and her goals in life. She had just sold her first painting when we saw her exhibit. Her art therapy process clearly connected her with both traditional and contemporary artists in China.

The energy of ink

Our intention was to create an opening for the conference that would combine Eastern and Western elements, with our American colleague, Music Therapist Krystal Demaine, MEd, MT-BC, playing guitar, Wang leading movement, and Gollub and Richardson planning the flow of movement onto paper.

As our group began to paint with the familiar Chinese materials (ink, bamboo brushes, and paper), the painted characters, lines, and images evoked smiles and laughter, and the flow of energy and feeling. In Wang's (in Richardson and Demaine, in press) words, movement makes "its mark in the heart and in the consciousness" as well as in visible form. Ink painting helps people to focus on their inner feelings, and their creative power. When the mark is made on paper, it is very easy to see the power and direction of movement. The understanding of the energy and direction in the art can then become an element for understanding the client and giving an accurate diagnosis for their present condition.

To the surprise of the Western therapists, as a first response to the artwork, Wang interpreted the images created by the flow of the ink, and related them to possible blockages in energy within the body and mind. This comment was a departure from our Western practice where therapists ask the clients to tell them about their artwork before reaching a diagnostic conclusion. Wang's interpretations connected to both the energy of the painting and the energy of the painter, in a context that was well understood by the group. Using art in diagnosis in this fashion, in the Chinese view, makes it easy to see the power and direction of the movement of energy, and the inner state of the artist. This state is mirrored in every brushstroke and line the artist or patient makes, whether in an image or in writing. According to Chou (2009), "In China, analyzing the structure of the character is a practice going back to antiquity" (p.187). In a parallel to Western art therapy theory, Cohen, Hammer and Singer (1988) discuss "line quality, line length and movement" (p.16) as three elements considered in analysis of drawings in the Diagnostic Drawing Series, a prominent Western assessment tool.

The American therapists were struck by how there is a holistic aspect to this way of looking at the myriad elements of art, and of diagnosis. We saw how the Chinese system of diagnosis carefully examines both the artwork and the overall situation of the individual, and looks at their functioning on many energetic levels. Wang cautioned us that it is important to see the relationship of the internal state of the person, and the external expression through art or language. An individual piece of art must be seen in the context of the inner response of the artist. The therapist can then become a guide to creating energetic movement and growth through art or movement. In Wang's approach, both therapists and clients use the materials of the creative arts to change the human spirit. Dance works with qi to bring awareness of space. Ink work visually records the power of qi on paper, and work with color works together with the imagination.

The movement of color and energy

Wang's work deepens awareness of the correspondences between the elements of art and the energetic state of the individual artist through her work with color. The different colors have particular meanings within the five element system, and working with color supports self-awareness and expression. While ink work makes people focus more on inner feeling, and their own creative power, work with color is more expansive in nature. This work is done within the context of the five elements, and particular colors can be used to strengthen certain elements. For example, after using blue, the addition of green may help people understand connections, such as the connection between water and the trees the water nurtures. After a young DaDance therapy client painted blue on his paper, he was helped to move to green by first doing a tree and grass growing dance improvisation. The dance movement helped balance his body by mobilizing his qi, and helping him to realize the driving force of life. Painting the movement made sure this awareness forever remained in his heart. As the ancient Chinese saying says, "A tree grows from the roots" (Reid, 1994, p.53), and this particular tree, the Taoist tree of health, is the foundation of all Traditional Chinese Medicine and work with energy.

Cane (1951/1983) used a strikingly similar exercise to help children gain "a little more courage, a little more freedom" (p.48). She chose to "suggest to the pupil that he is touching the ground and then reaching up towards the sky, or that he has a tree trunk between his hands, that he feels the trunk as he goes up and at the end he reaches out towards the tip of the branches" (p.48). Then she had him paint. Here again we noted Wang's connection with this pioneer of Western art therapy.

When working with a client, Wang works, as Cane did, with shifts between expressive modalities, from working with color to working with movement, to painting with ink. She also encompasses non-traditional media such as video; as when she used cartoons as a window to connecting with a reluctant eight-year-old boy with developmental delays. Working back and forth between a cartoon the child was fixated on, and the colors of the cartoon as painted on paper by Wang, she was finally able to engage his attention and to introduce color as a healing element. The picture created by the therapist became a focus of joint attention for the child and therapist, as they were increasingly able to explore the different colors together, and he became more responsive. He began making his own color choices to add to the process. The choice of color was, as always, a very significant element. As his initial choice, blue, became clear, his emotions became clearer as well. He became more cheerful and cooperative, and he began to show a greater interest in the picture created by the therapist. He became more invested in his own choices, more engaged, and increasingly responsive to others.

The participants in the conference, who included professionals, clients their parents, and students, also had an opportunity to experience the power of color in therapy firsthand in an experiential workshop with Wang. After warming up with movement, we each chose a color of brilliant tissue paper, and then relaxed with our color on the floor. The movement and relaxation experienced together encouraged us to go more deeply into our feeling state. Several of us chose a magenta color. This, we learned, was the color of the heart, the ruler of the five organ networks in the five element system. The heart connects to the flow of energy in the body, a vitally functioning organ, but one which is in danger of depleting the person's energy when it is overused emotionally. In the West, where there is no concept of the heart–mind, it is easy to put emotions in the heart, and easy to overwork the heart. Wang showed us that balance can be found through working with movement and art, and also by physical treatment to help wake up energy (Figure 4.3).

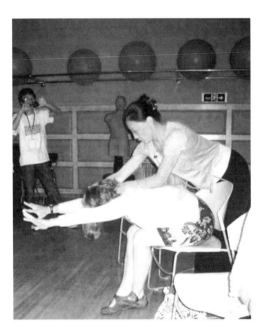

Figure 4.3 *Physical treatment after color exercise to mobilize qi*

Group energy provides a safe space

All through the conference, Wang moved our, by now, very eclectic group seamlessly through discussion to movement and art. She created the very same safe space we (Andrea and Jane) intended to explore in our workshop. This concept of safe space is one of the foundations of our Western approach to art therapy. We all seemed to understand the importance of safety in a similar way. Whether in Beijing or in the United States, the principles of creating safety are the same.

Our art therapy workshop became in some ways an extension of all the work we had done earlier. We visually and physically added the Western concept of containment by using small white paper boxes as the ground on which to create a personal safe space. We provided soft three-dimensional art materials to give a tactile feeling of safety and grounding. The most important element that we added was having participants share thoughts about their artwork with the group. Each artist had a chance to connect with and share their own inner world. This was done without interpretation.

Chinese and Western therapists met together to plan the details of the conference closing, which took place around a large sandtray. Wang's wish was to design an ending that would allow all conference members to go deep inside their hearts and minds and touch the human spirit. We decided to ask each member to bring to the sandtray their wishes and hopes for the future of the creative arts therapies in China. One participant constructed a Great Wall of China using glue sticks and sand which reflected her hope that we internationally bind together and build on the work we had shared.

The five elements and sharing our vision

As Wang articulated so beautifully for all of us, when we planned and experienced the ending sandtray, there was no division by nationality, but only our shared creation and intuitive understanding. As we created together in the sand there was a deep commitment from all to honor the concept of the five elements which were physically present in the sandtray: earth, present in the sand itself, the fire of a burning candle, and the images of metal and wood used for building our shared vision. The blue painted over the bottom of the sandtray represented water. In Chinese traditional culture, the best energy is like water!

Wang added multi-colored feathers to the tray because the feather is controlled by the lung, and the lung, in the five element system, is gold (or metal), and will give birth to water, helping to gather and integrate the positive energy of the different cultures. She shared her strong image with the group:

The most powerful water is flowing in the sandtray, makes the desert full of life with five powers. I see many people choose the images to try and tell a story. So I use the five color feathers to fill the soul and spirit. The feathers I use, red, blue, black, yellow and white, these are five colors that go with the power of spirit, soul, consciousness, ambition and energy. (Richardson and Demaine, in press)

In our work together we activated qi, or energy; and we also cultivated what McNiff (2009) calls "the vitality of the place" (p.166). Our shared experience made us all aware of how necessary and powerful the integration of Traditional Chinese Medicine and art therapy can be for developing practice in China.

References

Cane, F. (1983) *The Artist in Each of Us*, revised edn. Craftsbury Common, VT: Art Therapy Publications. (Originally published in 1951.)

Chou, H. (2009) *UCLA Chinese 187 Chinese Etymology and Calligraphy Course Reader Material*. Los Angeles, CA: Handout for course.

Cohen, B., Hammer, J. and Singer, S. (1988) "The Diagnostic Drawing Series: A systematic approach to art therapy evaluation and research." *The Arts in Psychotherapy 15*, 11–21.

Detri, K. (1983) "Foreword." In: F. Cane, *The Artist in Each of Us*, revised edn (p.iv). Craftsbury Common, VT: Art Therapy Publications.

Fu, J. (2009) "Chinese art of medicine and creative art therapy." *The Third Art and Natural Health Creative Art Therapy International Conference Journal*, 42–44.

Hearn, M. (2008) *How to Read Chinese Paintings*. New Haven, CT: Yale University.

McNiff, S. (2004) *Art Heals: How Creativity Heals the Soul*. Boston, MA: Shambhala.

McNiff, S. (2009) *Integrating the Arts in Therapy: History, Theory, Practice*. Springfield, IL: Charles C. Thomas.

Reid, D. (1994) *The Complete Book of Chinese Health and Healing: Guarding the Three Treasures*. Boston, MA: Shambhala.

Richardson, J. and Demaine, K. (in press) "The Arts and Natural Health: A Merging of Creative Arts Therapies and Traditional Chinese Medicine." In: S. Brooke (ed.) *The Use of the Creative Therapies Across Cultures*. Springfield, IL: Charles C. Thomas.

Sheng, H. (2011) *Fresh Ink: Ten Takes on Chinese Tradition*. Boston, MA: Museum of Fine Arts.

Sze, M. (ed.) (1992) *The Mustard Seed Garden Manual of Painting*. Princeton, NJ: Bollingen.

Van Briessen, F. (1998) *The Way of the Brush: Painting Techniques in China and Japan*. Rutland, VT: Charles E. Tuttle.

Wang, C. (2009) "The status quo and prospect of art therapy in China." *The Third Art and Natural Health Creative Art Therapy International Conference Journal*, 79–88.

Chapter 5

Towards an Integrated Medicine

Clinical Art Therapy in Korea

Sun Hyun Kim

Clinical art therapy is a new form of psychological treatment with art and medicine combined. It is understood as a method that evaluates and diagnoses the patient's physical and mental state and promotes disease treatment or symptom improvement through the art-making process. Clinical art therapy is based on the creative energy of art making. Other forms of the arts such as music, poetry, novels, and dance are also known to have therapeutic function. In the narrowest *sense*, clinical art therapy uses the art-making process of painting, carving, calligraphy, and craft making.

The most common inquiry about clinical art therapy is, "How can the art-making process offer disease-treating effects?" Clinical art therapy is not always a primary healing intervention like the direct treatment effects of how aspirin relieves a pain. Clinical art therapy offers healing within the framework of psychosomatic interrelations that primarily affects the mind. A complete genuine wellbeing is a state of overall achievement of physical, mental, emotional, social, and spiritual health. Since art making is a part of human nature—an integrative activity that comprehensively deals with physical, mental, emotional, social, and even spiritual factors— clinical art therapy can be considered as a secondary, indirect method to master the physical disease through mind stimulation and control the mind through stimulations to the body. The healing process can be said to be a creative process. Since the art activities of people are also a creative process in themselves, the creative process of the arts can lead directly to the healing of the body and mind. This means that acts of art can strengthen the natural healing power.

Voluntary art activities help individuals harmonize their internal and external wounds. Creating an art piece revitalizes the body and the mind, reduces stress, and increases healing capability. Art therapy is becoming the center of attention as a new alternative therapeutic model as part of the integrative medicine recognized throughout the world. There are various kinds of medical services in which art therapists work today, including preventive service, diagnostic evaluation, treatment, and assessment. In this chapter, I present the differences between Eastern and Western concepts of medicine to demonstrate how clinical art therapy can serve as a point of integration towards an integrated idea of health.

The differences between Eastern and Western medicine

Eastern and Western medicine both deal with human disease and each have their strengths. Western medicine has its strongpoint in surgical methods and is based on scientific research. Eastern medicine has proved its effectiveness in treatment (Jeon and Kim, 2009). Table 5.1 lists the differences of Eastern and Western medicine in basic philosophy and ideas.

Table 5.1 *The differences between Eastern and Western medicine*

Eastern medicine	Western medicine
Philosophical	Scientific
Subjective	Objective
Integrative	Analytic
Defensive	Aggressive
Experiential	Experimental
Humanistic	Technological
Holistic	Specialized
Adequate	Accurate
Orientated mind	Orientated diseases

Eastern medicine applies the Yin–Yang and Five Element Theory. This philosophical and metaphysical way of thinking is considered to be a comprehensive knowledge system. Meanwhile, Western medicine only includes those ideas confirmed through experiences and verifications. In essence, it is a system made up of unfinished knowledge. As a result, Western medicine emphasizes objective experiments and clinical outcomes. However, Eastern medicine considers the significance and importance of experience that has accumulated over thousands of years, allowing doctors to feel more comfortable making subjective judgments.

In terms of the cause of disease, Eastern medicine tends to attribute the problem to something related to the individual's overall system and therefore makes use of restorative herbal medicine for self-restoration. These medicines are uniquely prepared for patients to match their situations, as opposed to the mass production of identical tablets prescribed in the West. This type of treatment can be seen as quite passive and defensive when contrasted with the Western medicine assumption of disease as a result of a harmful foreign agent that invades the healthy body (Shea, 1992). This perspective calls for an active and aggressive regimen of blocking, eliminating, and removal. This difference may highlight why Eastern medicine doctors are trained more generally, whereas Western doctors tend to be specialists.

The two approaches also lead to different roles for doctors and patients. In Eastern medicine, the patient becomes the performer and the doctor is seen as an instructor in humanist medicine. It is common for doctors to provide assignments and responsibilities to patients. It is a similar relationship to athletes running in the field with their coach running beside them and giving instructions. Meanwhile, in technique-dependent medicine practiced in the West, patients are the beneficiaries and the doctor becomes the performer. Aside from taking medication, not many treatment duties are granted to the patient.

Psychotherapy and counseling in Korea

The different systems of medicine are not limited to physical health, but include the whole of a person, including mental health. The counseling culture is not familiar to the Korean population. The organized counseling system started in the US and therefore has been recognized as a product of American culture. In Korea, counseling officially started in 1985 when the Seoul Metropolitan Board of Education began counselor training. The development of counseling in Korea was marked by the adoption and application of the Western theories. However, efforts to develop counseling that suits the culture and character structure of Koreans have been made recently (Kim, 2006).

The Eastern and Western cultures greatly differ from their views of human nature (Table 5.2). Asians consider humans as a social and mutually dependent being. People who depend on others are caring, suppress themselves, and make concessions. The root of this view of human nature is to pursue modesty and harmony based on social identity. Meanwhile, the West sees a human as an individual and independent being and attaches great importance to active self-assertion, self-enhancement, competitions between individuals, and fair exchange. These differences in the view of nature and humans inevitably have an impact on the understanding and carrying out of psychotherapy. Understanding the self, self-transcendence beyond self-realization within relationships, and harmony are goals of psychotherapy in the East, while counseling in the West tends to stress individualism, self-realization, and self-satisfaction (Paloutzian, 1996).

Table 5.2 *Cultural differences in the East and West*

	East	West
Identity	Social identity	Personal identity
Culture	Collective culture	Individual culture
A view of nature	Change	Evolution
A view of relationship between human nature	Harmony	Struggle
Human relationship	Harmony and group-ism	Freedom and individualism
A goal of psychotherapy	Self-transcendence	Self-realization

One of the greatest cultural features of Korean people is "we-ness." The 2002 World Cup is a good example of the Korean nation showing their we-ness as the Korean peninsula was covered with Red Devils (Korean national football team), and became a role model to people throughout the world. Affection and resentment are emotions that represent the Korean nation. Affection is an integration of reason and emotion. According to *My Wife*, written by Kim Yoo-Jeong (2003), there is an expression "one feels more attached as we hate each other more, fight with each other more" (p.174). This is what Koreans often say as mixed feelings or detestable affection. Unlike the West where emotions and morality are ruled through reason, in the Korean psyche reason and emotions, even those that are contradictory, coexist (Hien and Honeyman, 2000).

A challenge to psychotherapy and counseling is that Korean people are generally not familiar or comfortable with revealing and expressing inner feelings, thoughts, or emotions. They consider the counselor as their teacher, tend to expect active counseling, and to cherish the self as a community being. The fear is that efforts therefore to correct oneself out of the context of the collective may lead to actions which may cause conflicts in the surrounding environment, the opposite of the valued harmony that is encouraged.

In order to prevent these collisions during counseling, a deep comprehension of the cultural differences between the East and West is required. When working with an individual, a clinician needs to begin with an understanding of the Korean culture and cultural characteristics and use it as a base line for understanding the interviewee's psychological state. For example, honor is a cultural feature of the Korean people. This characteristic is to not show one's true colors or act differently from the truth in order to enhance one's own or the opponent's position or prestige. It is an official self-image formed with values that are considered to be socially advisable. *Pansori*, an example of traditional Korean music, best reveals a Korean conception of resentment. Resentment is not revenge or showing one's frustration of desires or destructions in life; rather it is to suppress sorrow and release it through singing or dancing. The very nature of art therapy and its active use of the arts, as offering the possibility of nonverbal expression as a form of revealing an internal world, makes it compatible to the Korean psyche. Moreover, programs using the group feature, such as family art therapy and group art therapy, could be developed as a step towards developing a Korean art therapy.

Brief background and history of art therapy in Korea

Use of arts as a form of therapy can be traced as far back as ancient Korea, to the Buyeo Kingdom (2 bc–494 ad) and Goguryeo Dynasty (37 bc–668 ad). There are traces of art therapy that can be seen in historical Korean practices of art in ritual. Ancient tomb murals of the Goguryeo Dynasty brought treatment effects by recording the life of the deceased and expressing the wishes for the glorious life to be assured in the afterlife through art. The *Sashindo*, murals of four holy animals, also reflects the religious, integrated philosophy as the four holy animals are drawn in each direction to guard the tomb. Amulets and exorcism which still remain in our lives to this day are another form of art therapy and arts therapy. Amulets have voodoo effects with combinations of shapes and letters such as the sun, faces, and vortex expressed on paper to eradicate ghosts who bring ill health and bad fortune. These images are intended to counter these effects and bring good luck. A combination of art, dancing, music, and religious belief are applied in exorcism. Also, another source can be found in the application of the colors of five directions, which have been recognized as the basic colors of Korea, and in Yin–Yang and the Five Elements Theory.

Following the Korean War (1950–1953), psychiatry from the United States was officially introduced to Korea. Rather than replace traditional Korean ideas, there were attempts to integrate Korean culture and the philosophy of the Dao with a Western psychotherapy model (Garrity and Degelman, 1990). There were many skeptics who doubted the validity of this attempt, believing it to be a diversionary tactic in the name of art, rather than treatment by mental health professionals and psychotherapy specialists. Art therapy first started at Seoul National Hospital in 1960. However, art therapy at that time involved only art activities. Since then, art therapy in Korea has been developed by adopting Western-centered art therapy practices. After 1982, several more academic societies were established and since then interest in art therapy has grown rapidly. Nevertheless, the development has been by trial and error because there was no special agency or organization that could manage art therapy as a profession. Studies on the Eastern art therapy approach in Korea have been actively investigated in recent years (Jeon and Kim, 2009; Kim, 2006). The studies examine the Eastern movements centered on the areas, including counseling, medicine, art, and colors, and search for developing Eastern art therapy by combining the Eastern movements.

Common characteristics in therapeutic features of art therapy and Eastern medicine

Art therapy is compatible with Eastern medicine in many ways. Indeed it seems to be a natural fit, in line with the notions of health and illness, and as a result it has been pursued by a section of Korean clinicians as a part of enhancing medical treatment. As I have already mentioned, there are many differences between perceptions of health and illness, and medicine, between the East and the West, but art therapy seems to serve as a powerful bridge. In line with Korean medicine, art therapy begins with a health-centered notion. Art therapists work not only with patients with mental illnesses, but also ordinary people struggling with "unwellness." Art therapy has the potential to provide psychological stability and immunity improvement, and affects the entire human body in cancer patients, for example, or those undergoing rehabilitation with physical illnesses. This idea too can be found in Eastern medicine, which also recognizes the human body as a unified body.

Another bridge seems to be in the value placed on the accumulation of clinical experiences, in other words the acknowledgment of the whole. This means not only the value of health and illness, but also different types of treatment, which is the point from which Eastern medicine starts too. Lastly, it provides a bridge between being an active or passive patient. Both art therapy and Eastern, humanistic medicine includes the notion of the patient experiencing oneself being healed through creative processes.

The therapeutic concept of art therapy has not yet spread widely among the general population. Its limitations may be exceeded if a new concept is established by approaching the therapeutic and medical aspects of art therapy in the way of Eastern medicine.

Clinical art therapy as integrated medicine

Medicine in our times should be comprehensive, dealing with all areas of physical, mental, socio-psychological, and spiritual health beyond cultural boundaries. The phenomenon of alternative medicine is based on the needs that existing medicine does not manage health efficiently. The historical flow of medicine has shifted from "disease-oriented medicine" to "health-oriented medicine" in the 21st century. The axis has changed from "medicine for discovering and eliminating diseases" to "medicine promoting wellbeing." The physiological state of a person was divided into "health and disease" in the past due to quite relative and dichotomous ways of thinking. Now, we have a concept to describe the gray zone of "unhealthiness," which is the area between health and disease. The guardian of genuine health is one who dominates the area of "unhealthiness" and focuses on promoting wellness.

Clinical art therapy intervention can be seen as one of the most efficient treatment methods among the numerous complementary alternative medicines to comprehensively evaluate the patient's physical, psychological, social, and spiritual condition. It is still being researched as a complementary alternative intervention method. Clinical art therapy plays a role as an important part of complementary alternative medicine, and therefore has potential in the development of a holistic medicine. If we understand medicine in this way, doctors should be able to implement art therapy themselves. To do this, however, they need to be able to present rightful treatment courses and guidelines to their patients in their own areas by learning rightful research results and knowledge on art therapy.

For example, art therapy can offer clinical treatment to stroke patients, those suffering from paralysis, cognitive disorder, and arthritis, and cerebral palsy children within the rehabilitation medicine sector. It can also support the treatment of developmental disorder, learning disabilities, attention deficit hyperactivity disorder, autistic spectrum disorder, and children and families in the pediatric departments. Patients who are emotionally unstable, and those with social adjustment anxiety, depression, and other mental disease, could receive clinical help in the psychiatric area. Clinical art therapy can provide psychological stability with cancer patients, chronic pain patients, and those with other incurable diseases. In all of these areas, clinical interventions mean promoting the healing process of a disease.

Indeed clinical art therapy could contribute to the creation of a new world medicine. All medical models—Western, Eastern, and complementary alternative medicines—have their own strengths and have their limitations and weaknesses. If, however, the effectiveness of each of the medical models was integrated as a whole, a model of integrative medicine or holistic medicine of a class higher could be produced. Bringing Eastern art and Western medicine together, and ultimately harmonizing them into an Eastern–Western art and medicine, would give birth to a model of art therapy that is integrative and integrating. This area of integrative art therapy is expected to act as a catalyst in creating a new universal holistic medicine.

Conclusion

Today, clinical art therapy stands as a separate medical field supported through the cooperative relationship between various therapeutic specialists. At CHA University and Hospital, I have been expanding the clinical art therapy program into the medical center and hospital setting. This clinical art therapy model is managed through the cooperation of the clinic and the master's and PhD degree course in the graduate school. The medical center of CHA Hospital follows an integrated model that values a working relationship between Western medicine, Eastern medicine, and alternative medicine. The therapeutic modalities the CHA Hospital provides include acupuncture, homeopathy, clinical art therapy, neuro-feedback, body-work, chelation therapy, orthomolecular therapy, mind–body therapy, habit therapy, physiotherapy, intramuscular stimulation, neuro-linguistic programming, apitherapy, reconstructive therapy, cell therapy, and aesthetic therapy. It is within this context of integrative medicine that clinical art therapy plays an important role.

The goal of "opening up" is to help people understand the source of emotional distress or trauma and to alleviate and resolve conflicts. Opening up through art expression can also contribute to health and wellness, and sharing powerful or disturbing feelings is known to contribute to overall physical wellbeing. We are all familiar with the stressful effects of holding on to anger, anxiety, or grief. Unexpressed, these feelings can have harmful effects on the body, such as heart disease, chronic pain, or immune dysfunction. Research on the impact of expressing traumatic experiences underscores its health-giving benefits, including increased immunity and the need for fewer visits to a doctor (Malchiodi, 2006).

Art therapy in medical settings is practiced in hospitals, clinics, trauma units, and wellness centers. Medical applications of art therapy are a natural extension of the use of art therapy with psychiatric populations. The fundamental qualities that make the creative process empowering to children in general can be profoundly normalizing agents for those undergoing medical treatment. When the ill child engages in art making, he or she is in charge of the work—the materials to be used; the scope, intent, and imagery; when the piece is finished; and whether it will be retained or discarded. All these factors are under the child artist's control. Participating in creative work within the medical setting can help rebuild the young patient's sense of hope, self-esteem, autonomy, and competence while offering opportunities for safe and contained expression of feelings.

Art therapy has been used with a variety of pediatric medical populations, including those with cancer, kidney disease, juvenile rheumatoid arthritis, chronic pain, and severe burns. When medical art therapy is included as part of team treatment, art expression is used by young patients to communicate perceptions, needs, and wishes to art therapists, mental health professionals, child life specialists, and medical personnel. It is extremely useful in assessing each young patient's strengths, coping styles, and cognitive development. Information gathered through artworks can be invaluable to the medical team as it seeks to treat the whole person, not just the disease or diagnosis.

Acknowledgements

This chapter was informed by my collaboration with Dr. Douglas Degelman, Professor of Psychology, Vanguard University of Southern California.

References

Garrity, K. and Degelman, D. (1990) "Effect of server introduction on restaurant tipping." *Journal of Applied Social Psychology 20*, 168–172.

Hien, D. and Honeyman, T. (2000) "A closer look at the drug abuse–maternal aggression link." *Journal of Interpersonal Violence 15*, 503–522.

Jeon, S.I. and Kim, S.H. (2009) *Eastern and Western Medical Science and Eastern and Western Art Therapy*. Seoul: Hagjisa.

Kim, S.H. (2006) *Understanding Clinical Art Therapy*. Seoul: Hagjisa.

Kim, Y.J. (2003) *My Wife*. Seoul: Garam.

Malchiodi, C. (2006) *Art Therapy Sourcebook*. New York, NY: McGraw-Hill Contemporary.

Paloutzian, R.F. (1996) *Invitation to the Psychology of Religion*, 2nd edn. Boston: Allyn and Bacon.

Shea, J.D. (1992) "Religion and Sexual Adjustment." In: J.F. Schumaker (ed.) *Religion and Mental Health* (pp.70–84). New York, NY: Oxford University Press.

PART 2

Influence of Collectivism

Chapter 6

Collective Versus Individualist Societies and the Impact of Asian Values on Art Therapy in Singapore

Caroline Essame

Much of art therapy theory and practice has grown out of individualist Western societies and therefore naturally embraces many belief systems that characterize these societies. With the emergence of art therapy in Asia, however, where a more collective approach underpins society, a new era dawns rising with the Asian Tigers such as Singapore, Taiwan and South Korea, where the first Asian-based art therapy courses have been developed. This chapter will explore what questions may be asked to develop an Asian model of art therapy; what the relevant differences between Asia and the West are; and how to build on an understanding of art therapy when working with the variety of cultural, religious and socio-economic groups in Asia.

The terms West, East and Asia are highly contested. For the purposes of this chapter they will be used as shorthand to explore differences between different regions. It must be noted that Asia is far from homogeneous, but for the sake of brevity the term is used to account for an area and a mindset that may have significant differences from the dominant Western approach to art therapy. 'Asia' is used to describe the broad sweep from India to Japan. More specifically 'ASEAN' refers to the ten countries of the Association of Southeast Asian Nations where the word is used to focus more on the Confucian societies of South–east Asia, not including India, Sri Lanka and Pakistan, which do not share the Confucian background; and excluding China and Japan, which are large enough to be considered more valuably in separate terms.

One standard differentiation between Asia and the West is of collective versus individualist societies (Kim, 1995). That distinction helps our understanding of the two regions, but these terms should not be seen as mutually exclusive. This chapter considers that people behave in both collective and individualist ways, and operate within both frameworks to greater or lesser degrees. There is no dichotomy of the two; we are independent and part of a group at the same time. It is therefore valuable to see collective Asian values as complementary rather than counter to Western-style individualism.

As a result, this chapter looks not just at adapting art therapy to fit Asian values (outlined later), but also to consider it in a broader perspective than implied by Western individualism. Art therapy works with the social and emotional context of the individual; how the individual and group views and relates to the world around them gives art therapists the context for their work. Bearing this in mind, this chapter hopes to raise questions and broaden frameworks for art therapists in Asia as well as anyone working cross-culturally. Finally, it offers a suggestion for how art therapy might usefully incorporate lessons from Asia to be more inclusive across the world.

Asian values

When societies are collective, values are determined more by the group than the individual seeking their own way through the options of belief systems on offer. Everyone is influenced by the group in which they grow up, but in Asia the dominant values are held still to be of utmost importance for the individual. Not that there is homogeneity: in Southeast Asia, Confucian values and Christian values dominate in Singapore and Vietnam; Islamic values govern much social practice in Brunei Darussalam, Indonesia and Malaysia; Latin influences are widespread in the Philippines; and Cambodia, Laos, Myanmar and Thailand are steeped in Buddhist and Hindu values. But within this diversity there are core 'Asian values' that may be considered to reflect the collective spirit of this part of the world. According to the Bali Concord 11 as described by Ong (2003), an ASEAN citizen is characterized by a number of traits: family oriented, traditional minded, respectful of authority, consensus seeking, tolerant and sharing. Ng (2001), meanwhile, identifies six cultural characteristics that distinguish the culture of the East. Individuals are tightly organized, collective, hierarchical, place emphasis on social order and social harmony, possess a negative view of conflict and consider social approval important. To highlight how these ideas contrast with the West, the differences between individualist and collective societies are expanded in Table 6.1, which can help identify some of the fundamental and different belief systems for collective and individualist societies.

Table 6.1 *Differences between individuali and collective cultures*

Individualist	Collective
Independence from group	Interdependence with group
Independence as goal	Harmony as goal
Individuality in social settings	Conformity in social settings
Identity from unique traits/What *they* feel and express	Identity from place within the group/What others think
Aim for special recognition	Aim for understanding of group norms
Maintain opinions under attack	Change opinions for consensus
Concern with consistency	Concern with context
Monotheistic	Pluralistic

Adapted from Goncalo and Staw (2006)

Taking the basic social unit, the family, to illustrate these differences may help. Respect for elders and filial piety is a cornerstone of Asian values and reflects the hierarchical nature of most societies in Asia. In addition, as there is no welfare state, the family is commonly a more direct locus of support than may be the case in liberal Western countries. As a result, when verbal psychotherapy questions the role of the mother, it may challenge the honour and respect for elders – the filial piety. As a result, while it is difficult to confront parenting issues in a verbal way which would lead to uncomfortable and potentially damaging loss of face, it can be explored in greater safety using non-verbal arts therapies. The creative process does not necessarily need to be articulated verbally and a more developmental and non-analytical creative process framework can elicit profound change and resolution.

Western and Eastern values in art therapy

If asked what thoughts come to mind when given the three titles My Self, My Family and My Community, what would they be? And if asked to put these three titles in order of their influence on our lives, what would be the most influential aspect and which would be the least for the decisions that we make for our life and the social and emotional lens through which we judge and understand the world around us? This exercise establishes that there is a continuum from individualist to collective and everyone views the world with elements of the collective and the individualist and responds accordingly.

Much of Western health and social philosophy dates back to the Enlightenment and the 18th-century rise of liberal individualism that made personal rights of primary importance (Gombrich, 2005). In this context, the emphasis of the work of a therapist is often about ensuring that clients are able to live independent lives. This idea is reflected in the expectation that at age 18 children leave home and embark on a more individualist journey. It is also reflected in the pioneering notions of self-actualization and individualization (Freud, 1923/1996).

As described, this individual focus is far less common in Asia. As one example, children often stay with the extended families until they marry. Even then, they may move in with their in-laws once they marry, rather than live separate from family. Emphasizing this point in his Chinese New Year Speech, former Prime Minister of Singapore Goh Chok Tong (2004) outlined the balance of the collective, family and society with respect to the individual:

> Strong and stable families make for a strong and cohesive society… Singapore has to keep pace with developments in the world of ideas and learn from the West, but should not discard traditional values that make it a strong, close knit community…values like hard work, thrift, respect for elders and placing the community before self are the underpinnings of Singapore.

Increasingly, this Confucian ideal may be influenced by socio-economic and educational opportunities, such as families travelling abroad and the impact of globalization on cultural values. Still, the collective idea impacts profoundly on the Asian understanding in their interactions with their world and the life choices they make.

Identifying Asian values in Western theories

Even in the West, early therapists were looking at the individual in larger contexts. Beginning in the 1970s, Skynner (1987) pioneered systemic work by looking at the family in context, marking a move towards considering the individual within a collective. Many of the theories first explored by Jung (1961) have as much to contribute to art therapy in Asia as they have to existing Western-based training and practice. He described the personal and the collective unconscious, and much of his work grew out of looking at the beliefs and practices of East and West with the symbolism and archetypes that characterize these cultures. Exploring the work of Jung may therefore be a good place to begin to build a bridge between the Western and Asian models. His understanding of archetypes builds on Hindu and Buddhist philosophy, and his writing in the *Secret of the Golden Flower* (1967/1978) was based on the Chinese Taoist philosophy of the I Ching. Learmonth (1999) transposes these ideas in his exploration of Taoism and art therapy.

Defining the self

Rand (1957), the American writer and philosopher, sees man as a hero, with his own individual happiness being the moral purpose of his life; he exists for his own sake and should not sacrifice himself for others or indeed others for himself. This idea is reflected in the individualist concept of ego-strength, which is often used to describe the ability to know, feel and understand the self and how that self relates to the wider world. This idea was first defined by Freud (1923/1996) and may be described as the Western idea of the self. Yet when working cross-culturally, this basic concept comes under challenge. In different cultures, the definitions of self are varied. What do ego strength and the self mean in a collective context and how might this influence the way art therapists work?

Tu (1976) outlines how the Chinese concept of self is intrinsically linked to the collective, with its emphasis on the social need to care for others being inseparable from being true to oneself. He states that self-realization is innately connected to harmonizing human relations. Tu also explores how when a man marries and becomes a father only then is he considered a fully participating member of society. This approach offers key insights into what should be a core component of any Asian model; it is not about existing as an individual but rather a self deeply integrated with the group.

By way of further example, the Hindu concept of self as described in the Upanishads (Easwaran, 1987) sees self as part of the collective, spiritual and unattainable. The self is life, everywhere and indivisible, untouched by sin, and it is that self that holds the cosmos together. Marsella, Deros and Hsu (1985) describe the Hindu self as action-less, always attainable, formless, immutable and non-analytical. It is not identified specifically with the body, nor with intellect or cognition. Not an individual self, but a *dividual* self. In comparison they describe the Western self as analytical, monotheistic, individualist and rational. The difference is that in the West self is put *before* the collective and it is singular.

The Western way is to build the individual ego, which helps clients to be hospitable towards the group. From an Asian-values perspective we may be led to assume that, when the client feels good about the group, they will then grow in self-esteem. This idea would seem to suggest that any therapy model should work with the individual and the collective aspects of self as these are not an either/or dichotomy, but inform each other. When practising in Asia and working with individual ego development it is crucial to consider how an individual can function within a group. How individuals feel about themselves is intrinsically linked with how they will feel about other people. If they do not like themselves they are likely to feel hostile to others; if they feel good about who they are, they are more likely to be hospitable to others.

Harmony in relationships

This striving for harmonious relationships with others may be contrary to an assertive Western framework that encourages self-expression and considers that it is 'better out than in', and 'to thine own self be true', rather than the Chinese view 'to sacrifice the small me to complete the big me'. To illustrate the difference in these two approaches, in Confucian teaching, those who do not express their emotions are considered mature, wise and respectable, which a Freudian might define as being repressed. Weisz, Rothbaum and Blackburn (1984) further emphasize this idea in discussing that, in the West, yielding or giving in to emotions may be seen as a sign of weakness of character. In Confucian teaching, however, it reflects tolerance, flexibility, social maturity and particularly self-control. Inward self-control towards feelings and desires that might otherwise disturb interpersonal relationships shows the prized values of building harmony and maintaining *guan-xi* (relations) by giving and saving *mian-zi* (face).

The value put on the importance of hierarchies will also impact the early stages of establishing the therapeutic alliance. The therapist is immediately a figure of authority, an expert, and it is important the art becomes the medium, the avatar, and the therapist the holder of the space. The squiggle game is often a good ice-breaker, as used by Winnicott

(1971) and Thurow (1989) to set a level playing field and break down some of the expert/client dynamic. It gives the client permission to be playful and spontaneous and, as the therapist often makes the first mark in an open-ended way, it shows the client that there is no expectation to perform, no rights and wrongs in art making in this context.

Key components for an Asian model of art therapy

These Asian and Western beliefs can be seen on a continuum and, as the world becomes increasingly globalized and connected, people assimilate many different beliefs. What is striking about these comparisons is the different point from which these approaches start. For example, art therapists work with intuition, feelings and sensing of materials and encouraging clients to get in touch with spontaneous free expression. They may encounter additional challenges when the client gives priority to impulse control or what is thought rather than what is felt. The importance of being able to establish a trusting, accepting therapeutic relationship is paramount as it is only in this context that the therapist and the client will be able to work together and create a potential space (Winnicott, 1974), where growth and change can happen. Art as a visual and tangible medium provides a valuable third element to this relationship, and the third-person nature of the art making can help the client hold and explore what might be profound and unconscious processes that would not find a voice any other way.

There is a rich resource of stories, creativity and human experience coming out of the Asian region and it is exciting to be at the forefront of a new and different chapter in the history of art therapy and the healing arts. In response and summary to some of these questions and frameworks that have been explored, there are some key components to be considered for developing an Asian model of art therapy.

Non-analytical and less verbal approach

An understanding of hierarchies and face (*mian-zi*) may suggest working more non-verbally through the creative process and letting the art hold and carry the process while creating the therapeutic alliance and providing a safe, creative space. Where there is impulse control, the non-verbal nature of the creative process can be powerful and can transcend the cultural norms of the collective; the art is the third person, the metaphor for the experiences and life journey for the client. They can externalize and explore, and the unconscious processes of change and resolution take place without necessarily being owned directly and verbalized in a way that challenges cultural norms. If an individual feels safe in the therapeutic relationship he or she can work non-verbally and somehow, in the same way as the magic of play works in early childhood, bring internal change and resolution by making it visible, exploring it, taking control and then reintegrating it into the individualized self or indeed the collective self.

Group-orientated work: Considering interdependence and independence

When looking cross-culturally, the emphasis of therapeutic processes may differ in a Taoist or Confucian society where individualism is not prized in the same way as in a Western society. It is not uncommon for therapists in ASEAN countries to find parents referring their children to them with concerns for their group-socializing skills (collective) rather than their personal self-esteem and separation issues (individualist). What becomes clear is that these two areas are interlinked and inform each other. In clinical work with children, art therapy interventions may start as individual to build the therapeutic alliance and assess further the individual needs and processes, but the end aim may often be to integrate the client into a group.

Strong kinaesthetic component to work exploring mess and control

One recurring theme in working in art therapy in Singapore is the need to explore and work with mess (Beckerleg, 2009) and explore issues of control through this process. In societies where impulse control and pragmatic thought are prized above free expression and the understanding of feelings, what processes are in place that allow children and adults to explore and understand confusion and not knowing? When children play, they need to explore control of their external world through throwing toys, smearing paint, stacking, scribbling and all the other early childhood development processes that play therapists and creative arts therapists believe are so fundamental to the development of the ego (Essame, 2010; Jennings, 1999; Slade, 2001).

Often in individual and group sessions there is an intense realization that the child or adolescent needs to explore mess. In collective societies and particularly in Singapore and Hong Kong where most of the population live in small flats with little outside space, there is little scope or opportunity for messy play. Working large with wet paint, unconventional mark-making tools, clay and recycled rubbish gives these children a chance to explore and express many emotional states and intuitive processes over which they then feel some sense of control. They are not only told that they have to control their impulses, but they also learn how it feels and how it is processed and done through doing and feeling those processes and through creating their own order from them.

Encouraging the creative process

The great benefit of working with the visual arts, the third element in the therapeutic relationship, is that things can be processed through the tangible and physical experience of making art and the creations remain to be reviewed and revisited. The artworks over time have their own voice and the art therapist can help the client see the patterns, the movements, the journey personified through the art. As the therapist holds the safe space, the art medium and the processes of engaging in creating can help the client along a journey in which they can explore, and perhaps even be surprised and change. The power of art is its potential to express metaphorical life experiences of the conscious and unconscious, the individual and collective, through the creative process.

I have particular experience in this area with children with special needs who because of their processing challenges are not able to develop and understand the social needs and norms of the group. When working with children on the autistic spectrum, this need for exploring and developing spontaneity, creativity and imagination, and understanding the control of these processes, becomes very obvious. If the child has not explored them at their developmental stage, there are few later opportunities available to them. The nature of art making in a therapy context offers an invaluable sensory, physical, emotional and tangible experience for them that they might otherwise never receive (Beckerleg, 2009; Martin, 2009).

Educating the caregiver on the role of play and creativity

It is often important to expose the family to an understanding of the role of creativity in human development. We need to bear in mind that many children in Asia are raised by extended families or other caregivers. In art therapy, the nature of the therapeutic alliance is as fundamental to the process of growth and change as the engagement in art making. It is part of the three-way alchemical relationship that makes art therapy so powerful. The importance of a nurturing, empathic relationship in early childhood (Greenspan and Shanker, 2004; Greenspan and Wieder, 2006; Kravits, 2008) needs to be explored and understood in the context of Asian societies. There is much scope for dialogue and education for parents, domestic helpers and early childhood educators on how to nurture and provide that creative potential space where ego, both collective and individual, can be developed and explored through play and creativity.

Conclusion

This chapter has highlighted how collective and individualist societies may approach their personal and group understandings of the world. An Asian model of art therapy will hopefully add to the broad spectrum of art therapy approaches and models that developed from the West. The nature of the art therapy process with its emphasis on the therapeutic relationship, kinaesthetic effects of art making and emphasis on creativity has begun a new journey in Asia. As with any creative journey this integration should lead to growth and new perspectives in the field.

References

Beckerleg, T. (2009) *Fun with Messy Play: Ideas and Activities for Children with Special Needs.* London: Jessica Kingsley Publishers.

Easwaran, E. (1987) *The Upanishads.* London: Penguin Arkana.

Essame, C. (2010) 'Understanding art making from an art therapy perspective.' *International Art in Early Childhood Research Journal 2,* 1. Available at www.artinearlychildhood. org/artec/images/article/ARTEC_2010_Research_Journal_1_Article_7.pdf, accessed on 2 March 2012.

Freud, S. (1996) In: J. Strachey (ed.) *The Complete Psychological Works of Sigmund Freud* (p. XIX). London: Hogarth. (Originally published in 1923.)

Goh, C.T. (2004) 'Chinese New Year Speech.' Available at http://stars.nhb.gov.sg/stars/ tmp/PM-GohChokTong-CNY-Message-2004.pdf, accessed on 4 November 2011.

Goncalo, J.A. and Staw, B.M. (2006) 'Individualism-collectivism and group creativity.' *Organizational Behavior and Human Decision Processes 100,* 96–109.

Gombrich, E.H. (2005) *A Little History of the World.* New Haven, CT: Yale University Press.

Greenspan, S. and Shanker, S. (2004) *The First Idea: How Symbols, Language and Intelligence Evolved from Early Primates to Modern Humans.* Cambridge, MA: Da Capo Press.

Greenspan, S. and Wieder, S. (2006) *Infant and Early Childhood Mental Health.* Washington DC: American Psychiatric Publishing.

Jennings, S. (1999) *Introduction to Developmental Play Therapy: Playing and Health*. London: Jessica Kingsley Publishers.

Jung, C.G. (1961) *Memories, Dreams and Reflections*. New York, NY: Random House.

Jung, C.G. (1978) 'Commentary on "The Secret of the Golden Flower".' In: *Psychology and the East* (trans. R.F.C. Hull). Princeton: Princeton University Press. (First published in 1967.)

Kim, U. (1995) *Individualism and Collectivism: A Psychological, Cultural and Ecological Analysis*. Copenhagen: NIAS Publications.

Kravits, K. (2008) 'The Neurobiology of Relatedness: Attachment.' In: N. Hass-Cohen and R. Carr (eds) *Art Therapy and Clinical Neuroscience* (pp.131–146). London: Jessica Kingsley Publishers.

Learmonth, M. (1999) 'Taoism and Art Therapy, Flowing and Stuckness.' In: J. Campbell, M. Liebmann, F. Brooks, J. Jones and C. Ward (eds) *Art Therapy, Race and Culture* (pp.192–208). London: Jessica Kingsley Publishers.

Marsella, A., Deros, G. and Hsu, F. (1985) *Culture and Self – Asian and Western Perspectives*. London: Tavistock.

Martin, N. (2009) *Art as an Early Intervention Tool for Children with Autism*. London: Jessica Kingsley Publishers.

Ng, A.K. (2001) *Why Asians are Less Creative than Westerners*. Singapore: Prentice Hall.

Ong, K.Y. (2003) *ASEAN Cultural Connections: ASEAN Values and its Relevance to the Modern World*. Unpublished opening address by Secretary General of ASEAN at ASEAN Cultural Connection Seminar, Singapore, 12 November 2003. Available at www.aseansec.org/15988.htm, accessed on 4 November 2011.

Rand, A. (1957) *Appendix: Atlas Shrugged*. New York, NY: Random House.

Skynner, R. (1987) *Explorations with Families: Group Analysis and Family Therapy*. London: Tavistock/Routledge.

Slade, P. (2001) *Child Play – Its Importance in Human Development*. London: Jessica Kingsley Publishers.

Thurow, J. (1989) 'Interactional squiggle drawings with children: An illustration of the therapeutic change process.' *The Focusing Folio 8*, 4, 149–186.

Tu, W.M. (1976) 'The Confucian perception of adulthood.' *Daedalus 105*, 2, 109–123.

Weisz, J.R., Rothbaum, F.M. and Blackburn, T.C. (1984) 'Standing out and standing in: The psychology of control in America and Japan.' *American Psychologist 39*, 955–969.

Winnicott, D.W. (1971) *Therapeutic Consultations in Child Psychiatry*. New York, NY: Basic Books.

Winnicott, D.W. (1974) *Playing and Reality*. London: Pelican Books.

Chapter 7

Understanding of Korean Culture and the Value of the Art Therapeutic Approach

Lee Min Jung

The focus of this chapter is on examining the benefits of art therapy for children with disabilities in Korea. Art therapy may be particularly helpful given its role in addressing limitations of expression, lack of communication, and difficulties with social skills. I will also address how art therapy can be offered in a manner that is in accordance with Korean values and family structure.

Korean family values

When one ethnicity remains homogeneous for a long time, a common lifestyle is established and reinforced. Even though it may vary over time, its fundamental spirit remains the same and creates a nation's own unique living culture (Lee *et al.*, 2009). Traditionally, Korean society is based on Confucian ideas, which have been internalized in the individual's daily life to such an extent that it is often taken for granted as unquestionable and correct behavior. The two axes of Confucian society are family and nation. Family is the most basic unit that forms society in a vast country, and is an initial unit of social life where people learn interpersonal skills through parent–child, sibling, and marital relationships. It is the family that constitutes the core of the organizational system in all aspects (Kum, 1989) and is responsible for ensuring that cultural values are acquired and transmitted. An individual's lifestyle is determined by the family. The importance of the family can be understood as a historical accumulation of social experiences with characteristics that connect many generations. Given that there are certain limits in the larger society of the extent to which a certain attitude, value system, opinion, interest, and specific activity can be accepted, individual lifestyle can be influenced by socially accepted standards as transmitted through the family. As people live together, they construct a group identity. However, each family culture is relative within one ethnicity, demonstrating its own unique differences (Song, Lee and Jung, 2009). In Korean society, the family culture shows a strong homogeneous element, but the degree of adherence to societal expectations may be different for each family and each family member.

Even while adhering to traditional values, Koreans have observed a reconfiguration and reconstruction of the family as a system (Kim, 1997). Traditional values may or may not match the rapidly changing reality. The discrepancy between traditional and new attitudes and values often leads to conflicts in family relationships and between generations. As an example, parent–child communication has become more difficult due to changing living patterns between parents and children and the gap between their values, specifically in how to identify solutions to remedy family problems. Parents who value traditional Korean culture and privilege the Confucian family lifestyle are bound to have cultural and lifestyle differences, with children greatly affected by the inrush of Western culture and its emphasis on the private-driven life. Encouraged by mass media or the internet, younger Koreans are actively embracing foreign culture, and are entering an era marked by an emphasis on individuality. Meanwhile, parents who preserve and pass along traditional values are hitting the limits of their understanding and acceptance of the values and culture of their children. As an outgrowth of the increased emphasis on personal desires and individual needs, family life is also changing. The individual is increasingly put first as the culture moves away from family-centric thinking.

Still, the family culture influences the behavior and emotions of individual family members, performing an important socialization function (Norlin and Chess, 1997). Koreans learn how to regulate their values and behaviors according to specific rules and constraints learned in childhood. For example, most Koreans learn that we must be careful not to insist on the self, saying "our house" or "our family" rather than "my house" or "my family." This preference for plural possessive adjectives reflects the collectivist values of Korea, imposed to ensure harmony and maintain balance within the family and society (Nisbett, 2004). This value system is maintained under the belief that children are bound to parents by virtue of having come from the same ancestors.

Since family in Confucianism is the essential element in structure of Korean society, it is not something that belongs only in the era in which we live. Rather, it has been recognized as an eternal institution that has been descended from our ancestors and will be inherited by our descendants. If the family is unstable, all of the members, including children, risk having various problems. As a result, most Korean families still consider the value of managing and maintaining homes as a central core value. The family is a source of happiness and welfare, leading many to be hesitant to admit or quick to deny that it can be the source of problems. Since expressing or asking for outside help for family problems is viewed as shameful or dishonorable, many attempt to resolve conflicts within the family. This point reveals that the family can also be the starting point of solving problems.

It is necessary to define the role of expression in identifying the causes of conflicts in the home. In this chapter, *expression* refers to the act of freely sharing one's thoughts and opinions, as well as the ability to form relationships with others and maintain communication with them. Children learn appropriate communication methods from family and how to decide who they can share their thoughts or ideas with so as to foster good family relationships, friendships, and social relations that enhance their ability to minimize conflicts and problems, and ensure harmony. Despite obvious differences among family members, they share everything within the family, and learn from their parents' traditional methods of communication. The Confucian vertical family structure of Korea is focused on discipline, sacrifice, and temperance, which places an emphasis more on the result than the process. At times this expectation means that the emotions need to be suppressed, and that there is little place for the expression of feelings. When individuals do not express their desires or intentions for fear of being rejected by others because of negative emotions, or do not recognize their own feelings by excessively suppressing their feelings or thoughts, individuals may experience internal tension that can interfere with sustaining and developing secure family relationships (Song *et al.*, 2009). Therefore it has been recognized that open communication can lead to stable and intimate relationships, as well as increased problem-solving abilities, demonstrating how free expression can be an important element in healthy ego development, mental health, and sociality of children (Ministry of Gender Equality and Family, 2010).

Accessing treatment services in Korea

It remains difficult for Koreans to recognize their own problems and ask others for help or take action to share their stories or those of their family with strangers, even to resolve conflicts within the family. It is reasonable to seek professional counseling or therapy when necessary, and where possible, to benefit from a variety of social welfare services provided by the government. However, although many recognize the need for such measures, a prejudice against receiving treatment services remains, since Koreans are sensitive to how others view them, striving to make not "I" but the "view on me" the subject. As a result, distribution and accessing of necessary social services is limited. Thus, even though we have applied various social welfare service models derived from the practice of the US and Europe to Korean society, the execution of those initiatives has been beset by limitations.

The welfare system in Korea is overburdened, which leads to great difficulty in securing sufficient professional staff for treatment services. Social welfare services typically emphasize the quantitative aspect of numbers served instead of the qualitative aspect related to care. Additionally, the welfare services on a national level do not include post-treatment services aimed at continuity of care and maintenance. The service providers focus on treating past and current problems, rather than offering preventive services in response to personal disorders and various problems that occur within a family (Kim, 1997). Given that many families in Korea already do not discuss problems or perceive tensions as problems, the lack of preventive services leads to greater difficulties in resolving family tension.

Investment and expertise in the therapeutic arena and in training and dissemination are still in development. Although an awareness of the importance and value of therapy services is spreading, few hospitals or centers are able to hire therapists. Additionally, the relatively small percentage of hospital professional staff who provide welfare services makes it difficult to find treatment specialists (National Assembly Budget Office, 2007). The South Korean system is also beset by unclear definitions concerning therapist qualifications. Treatment services are often offered by privately certified therapists, under a relative absence of government registration or recognition. Strict, unified criteria for qualifying therapists have not been legally established in Korea (Kim, 2009). The presence of unqualified therapists and the lack of a system to regulate them are pressing problems that directly impact the quality of health services. As users are free to select their preferred service provider, the differences among professionals affect client satisfaction level (Seo and Min, 2010).

Because access to Korea's welfare system is limited to the lower class, people experience shame associated with receiving welfare-related treatment services. Those receiving welfare services are a diverse population, but among them there is a growing need of services for children with developmental disabilities. Complicating this need is a general negative perception of and prejudice against people with disabilities in Korean society. Because children with disabilities evince a range of problems related to intelligence, emotional control, communication, behavior, and sociability, they often require special education in addition to treatment services.

Art therapy within art education

Among the services that children with disabilities receive, they often prefer art making. Fortunately, it also promotes healthy development in children by stimulating sensory, emotional, and social areas, thereby promoting holistic growth (Lee and Choi, 2008). As a result, art has been applied actively in educational and treatment settings (Rubin, 2005). In Korea, the acceptance of art therapy services for children with disabilities is increasing in hospitals, as well as in therapy centers and various educational institutions. Since art itself has benefits that allow for natural interactions and non-verbal communication, it has been widely integrated and used to enhance the therapeutic effect. Typically, services for children with disabilities have consisted of some form of special education. These programs contain courses focused on providing basic functional life training to allow them to lead independent and productive lives, while also complementing cognitive and social deficits. As the importance of educational and care services are introduced to people with disabilities, needs and requirements have increased (Park et al., 2008). Art activities are being recognized for their importance in treatment and potential to transcend a purely educational stance (Lee and Choi, 2003).

In special education settings, art therapy integrated into art education provides the therapeutic aspects that can overcome psychological conflicts and behavior problems resulting from disabilities and allows for the necessary accommodation required for children of various disability levels (Henley, 1992). Although art itself is useful, for children with disabilities there are limitations to its benefit if not offered within the context of art therapy. Art therapy in a therapeutic education setting is offered in art classes that are clearly distinguished from general art education and the art teaching method. One of the ways it differs from art education is that it is tailored to the individual's disabilities and encourages openness and autonomy in teaching methods through exploring media and artistic activities. The educational approach to art therapy for children with disabilities is a way for them to experience their inner world and improve their socialization.

Art therapy with children with disabilities

Through art therapy, children with disabilities show improvement in sensory integration and emotional expression through non-verbal and symbolic representations that stimulate the possibilities of other communication (Kim, 2010). Art therapy can be an effective means of self-expression compared to traditional verbal therapy, since it is a communication tool that children commonly prefer. Aside from aiding the direct effects of the disabilities, children with disabilities often have accompanying psycho-social problems, such as low self-esteem, which can manifest as various socially maladaptive behaviors (Lee and Choi, 2003). As art is an active and voluntary form of self-expression, it can help children with disabilities transcend limited abilities and structured environments to establish social relationships and enhance their educational experiences.

For children with ADHD, a structured environment and framework may reduce distraction and impulsive tendencies. Without proper regulation and control by the therapist, there can be too much stimulation in the treatment environment, resulting in the child having difficulty in paying attention. The therapist would do well to create an activity that requires completing a directive sequentially and presenting media to stimulate curiosity. In that way, the child will be able to increase his or her attention span, deploy more systematic activity, and grow task performance skills on an ongoing basis as he or she applies a great deal of energy to accomplishing tasks (Henley, 1998).

Through group art therapy, children listen to each other's ideas and opinions. As children express themselves more freely and touch on topics that were hard for them to share, they come to perceive that both the art therapist and the group members can begin to understand their problems. They subsequently seem more able to show their feelings and emotions around these topics. In addition, they become empowered to search for solutions individually and collectively to resolve their psychological conflicts and dissatisfactions they previously could not reveal.

Children with cognitive delays, sensory integration difficulties, limitations on physical ability, and impaired language skills have limited opportunities to establish relationships and express their needs. Like all humans, these children are social beings who evolve in relationship with others. When relationships with others are amicable and harmonious, people can grow into well-adjusted adults. Interpersonal relationships significantly influence children's social, cognitive, and emotional development (Kim, 2010). For this development to take place, children need to express appropriately their emotions and require the freedom to practice communicating their desires and problems. However, Korean children's ability to reveal their feelings and relieve their stress can be limited. Sometimes these limitations are those of opportunity; at other times they are a result of cultural family norms; but sometimes expression is hampered by a lack of knowledge concerning how to express. In this regard, art becomes a non-verbal means of stimulating such expression. Children communicate with their environment or world, and themselves, through art. Using art, children communicate with others, while creating an environment that allows them to share their thoughts or feelings with others. Above all, their own creations allow them an outlet to communicate with themselves. They look back upon or reveal themselves through this process, and come to understand others better through their own artistic expression (Lee et al., 2008).

In order to meet the demands and needs for such opportunities, art therapy can be aimed at developing children's awareness, emotional expression, and behavior, as well as enhancing the mental and social functions that impact academic performance and emotional functioning. Additionally, they mirror cultural norms aimed at fostering relationships. In group art therapy for children with disabilities, art therapists should create the optimal program by considering the characteristics of the group including disability and degree of development. They then need to select features that maximize social improvement by carefully paying attention to how the technical and expressive aspects of art making can enhance natural interactions between group members. Two important areas that art therapists can target are in the use of art for communication and in the development of social skills.

Art therapy to enhance communication

Children with disabilities suffer the pain of their limitations, feelings of inadequacy, and isolation. These feelings are impacted by their difficulty maintaining and developing relationships, related to a lack of empathy, other awareness, and appropriate communication skills for sharing their thoughts (Berry and Marshal, 1978). For children who have problems in expressive aspects of language, art therapy helps them share their problems or conditions, and moreover it gives them the opportunity to increase their self-esteem by showing their strengths and aiding their socialization. Children have a fundamental desire to express themselves through their own unique ways, and are born with basic abilities for expressing themselves using visual images, just as they represent themselves in spoken language. Art therapy as non-verbal communication allows children who are not otherwise free to express themselves because of a lack of linguistic expression ability to utilize images to express problems, conflicts, feelings, and thoughts more freely by combining scribbling, drawing, and various media.

The sculptures in Figure 7.1 were created by two brothers in art therapy who were referred for distracting behaviors, lack of control, and aggressive words and actions. After their parents divorced, they grew up with their mother and stepfather, but because proper discipline and care was not maintained, they felt very insecure psychologically. The older brother was unable to focus on a given activity or sit still, wandering around the therapy room. In contrast, the younger child evinced a liking of art, showed curiosity about the materials, and tried to complete the piece he was working on. As the family stories were disclosed, the child was able to express his emotions, dissatisfactions, and hopes. The younger child gave his older brother materials so he could participate in the activities, and also tried to motivate him through showing what he had made. As a result, the older brother began to use the same materials his younger brother was using, creating a masterpiece in another form. When the subject turned to family, he also shared his negative feelings with his younger brother.

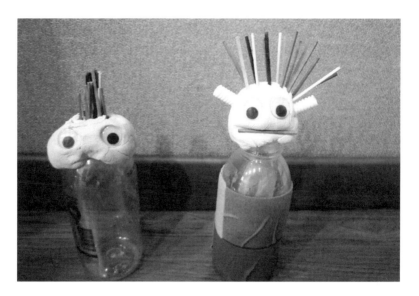

Figure 7.1 *Two brothers' sculptures*

Through art therapy, the children received the opportunity to open their hearts and share their unexpressed emotions and dissatisfactory experiences. In addition to learning how to express themselves, they were also able to strengthen their sibling bond, thus reinforcing the importance of family. The sessions demonstrated how art therapy can simultaneously support family relationships, while permitting continuous communication to better understand their own problems and search for positive solutions.

Art therapy to enhance social skills

People need social skills to interact successfully with peers and to adapt to their environments. Children with disabilities show impairments in social functioning, which are reinforced through limited social interactions. Impaired social skills may also be a result of peer rejection due to a propensity to angry explosions or hyperactivity. Both may be due to difficulties controlling anger and aggressive behavior. Children who have been repeatedly neglected by peers may exhibit shyness and social reluctance (Cho, 1998).

　　Art therapy groups are effective because they provide a therapeutic environment where children can stop feeling reluctant about social limits by sharing their opinions with others and exercising autonomy. Children in art therapy will naturally experience relationships by sharing art supplies or complimenting each other's drawings. Moreover, people have the opportunity to exchange information in group art therapy by talking about their drawings and experiences with each other. They will have an opportunity to learn new things and teach at the same time, while imitating others' behaviors. Art therapists can help members learn various social techniques by sharing mutual feedback. The group members will be able to learn better interpersonal relationships while changing out distorted feelings and thoughts. This interpersonal learning allows children with disabilities to develop their ability to control their expressions due to the structure of the group rules, which foster expression of their opinions and feelings. These improvements allow them to get closer with other group members and to develop a sense of community by forming positive relationships. To maximize these benefits, group art therapists may want to create groups with children with a range of social functions and disability levels, so that children with disabilities can improve their social skills by taking advantages of group dynamics.

Figures 7.2 and 7.3 show the work of a child who was referred based on having a number of difficulties in peer relationships and a variety of social problems. She didn't like the therapist intervening in her work, and even when the therapist tried to ask questions or hold a conversation, she answered briefly or showed that she just wanted to continue what she wanted to do, virtually ignoring the therapist. However, beginning with the fourth session, through the "making a friend project," she expressed a desire to make friends symbolically in the form of insects. She also began to create joint spaces where she and her friends could live together. Through this process, she was able to create various situations, envisioning how she could start to make friends, cope with matters when there were conflicts with them, and how she could tune her opinions with those of others. In that creative process, it was possible for her to learn to acquire the peer relationships and social skills a child needs. Additionally, through naturally sharing her private thoughts, emotions, and experiences with the art therapist, she was able to ask for advice, and eventually even invited help in her work. Moreover, through parent therapy sessions, it was possible to create an environment at home in which the parents could adopt a stance, so that she could share her concerns, while they looked for various solutions. The client was able to acquire social techniques to help her address various conflicts and problems that can occur with peers, and the family was provided with a set of strategies for maintaining peace in the home.

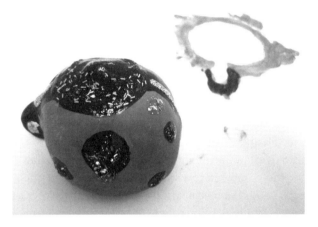

Figure 7.2 *Symbolic friend (1)*

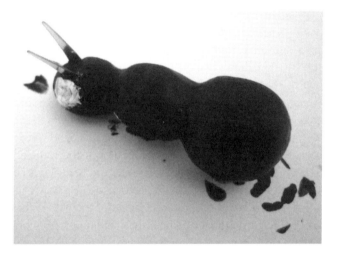

Figure 7.3 *Symbolic friend (2)*

Conclusion

In order to understand Korean society, it is important to understand how "I" as a member of the family has been sacrificed and suppressed for the maintenance and peace of the family. To support individuals while honoring the family, I have found that offering services within regular settings, such as schools, provides a balance of Western ideas of therapeutic expression with Korean values. In particular, art therapy is an excellent method, serving as a new language for children with disabilities. As seen in the case examples and from other children I have worked with in art therapy, they have been able to radiate feelings formerly repressed as a result of their difficulty expressing things in language and the societal taboos on sharing negative emotions. For them, art has become an important medium for social interaction. Additionally, it is becoming an excellent tool when used in conjunction with special education and art education. Through art therapy, people are able to reset emotional conflicts and unsatisfactory situations in their lives, express their emotions or thoughts naturally, and reach resolutions on their own.

References

Berry, P. and Marshal, B. (1978) "Social interaction and communication pattern in mentally retarded children." *American Journal of Mental Deficiency 25*, 2, 44–51.

Cho, Y.T. (1998) "Developmental trend in social skill of mentally retarded children." *Journal of Developmental Disabilities 2*, 43–54.

Henley, D. (1992) *Exceptional Children, Exceptional Art: Teaching Art to Special Needs.* Worcester: Davis Publications.

Henley, D. (1998) "Art therapy in a socialization program for children with Attention Deficit Hyperactivity Disorder." *American Jounral of Art Therapy 37*, 1, 2–12.

Kim, H.S. (2010) *The Effects of the Photorealism Art Therapy Education Program on The Social Skills in Children with Developmental Disabilities.* MA dissertation, Daegu, Korea: Daegu University.

Kim, M.D. (1997) "Changes of Korean family in 21st century and social welfare measures." *Korea Institute of Family Social Work 2*, 11–30.

Kim, S.H. (2009) "Art therapy development in Korea: The current climate." *The Arts in Psychotherapy 36*, 1–4.

Kum, J.T. (1989) *Understanding Korean Confucianism.* Seoul, Korea: Bookpia.

Lee, G.M. and Choi, I.H. (2008) *Practice of Art Therapy through Media Experience.* Seoul, Korea: Sigma Press.

Lee, G.M. and Choi, W.S. (2003) *Practice of Art Therapy in Helping Infantile and Child Development.* Kyung-Gi, Korea: Gyoyook Books.

Lee, G.S., Kim, D.Y., Ryu, J.M., Jeon, S.S. *et al.* (2008) *Art Education.* Kyung-Gi, Korea: Gyoyook Books.

Lee, J.W., Gae, S.J., Yang, S.H., Lee, Y.S. and Park, M.S. (2009) *Family and Culture.* Seoul, Korea: Sin Jung.

Ministry of Gender Equality and Family (2010) *The 2nd National Survey of Korea's Families.* Seoul, Korea: Ministry of Gender Equality and Family.

National Assembly Budget Office (2007) *Budget Analysis of 2008 (III).* Seoul, Korea: National Assembly Budget Office.

Nisbett, R. (2004) *The Geography of Thought: How Asians and Westerners Think Differently… and Why.* New York, NY: The Free Press.

Norlin, J.M. and Chess, W.A. (1997) *Human Behavior and the Social Environment: Social Systems Theory.* Boston, MA: Allyn and Bacon.

Park, E.H., Kim, M.S., Kim, S.J., Kang, H.K. *et al.* (2008) *Art Education for Children with Disabilities.* Seoul, Korea: Hakjisa.

Rubin, J.A. (2005) *Child Art Therapy.* New York, NY: Wiley & Sons.

Seo, D.M. and Min, S.H. (2010) "A study on the method for the development of the rehabilitation service for the disabled children." *Journal of Disability and Welfare 2,* 75–93.

Song, J.E., Lee, Y.H. and Jung, H.E. (2009) *Family and Life Culture.* Seoul, Korea: Yang Seo Won.

Chapter 8

The Life Garden Project Art Therapy Intervention for Depressed Elderly in Hong Kong

A Communal Support Approach

Julia Byrne

This chapter highlights the positive impact of the Art Therapy Groups of the Life Garden Project. This three-year therapeutic endeavour from 2006 to 2009 integrated a range of holistic therapy interventions, in a concerted effort to reduce depression levels for 200 elderly living in the New Territories of Hong Kong.

I will begin with a background of the group members including a historical lens highlighting the impact of migrating to Hong Kong from mainland China and the challenges of sustaining traditional Chinese customs and belief systems for the Hong Kong elderly, one of which is the loss of communal living. Next, I will present the framework of the art therapy groups of Life Garden, which emphasized the sense of communal living as a way to re-integrate communal support and traditional Chinese values to enhance the healthy emotional functioning for this generation of Hong Kong Chinese elderly.

Background of Life Garden Group members

On the whole, elderly people in Hong Kong today have faced a lifetime of struggles beginning in childhood. The majority of the group members with whom I worked were born in mainland China, largely from the rural areas of the southern region, and lived there throughout their early years. Many migrated to Hong Kong during the early to mid 1950s as children or adolescents, during one of the largest influxes of refugees from the mainland, crossing the border into Hong Kong in the midst of the Nationalist–Communist Civil War.

The economic climate in Hong Kong was weak during this time with a plethora of people facing impoverishment, lack of jobs, limited resources and still recovering from Japanese occupation, which ended in 1945. There was a huge swell in population, rising to 2.2 million by the early 1950s, making Hong Kong one of the most densely populated cities in the world. The administration struggled to accommodate these immigrants, and the newcomers erected shacks for their homes using any material available, or had to settle for cramped quarters (Welsh, 1997). This generation of immigrants also faced certain cross-cultural barriers. Although Hong Kong and mainland China share the same Chinese traditions, they have different ways of expressing them. An important difference was in the communal living system that was deeply engrained in the mainland and in their lives, but was unable to be actualized in Hong Kong, due to their being separated from their extended families and support systems. In addition, they had to adapt to temporary living conditions, overcrowding and lack of employment. The elderly of today worked hard to create a better life for themselves and their families in their adult years, with the majority of them working for little pay in farming and fisheries, as tailors and in the service industry.

Elderly Chinese and depression in Hong Kong

Hong Kong today is facing an ever-increasing ageing population. Elderly depression is a growing concern and a major public health problem, which has a considerable impact on both individuals and society (Chan et al., 2006). In 2006, when the Life Garden Project began, there were 6,864,346 people in Hong Kong. The number of those aged 65 and over were 852,796 or 12.4 per cent of the elderly population (Census and Statistics Department, 2011). Over 5 per cent of the total elderly population were diagnosed with depression (Census and Statistics Department, 2006).

In Woo, Ho and Lau's study (as cited in Shetye, 2007) risk factors contributing to depression for elderly Chinese in Hong Kong were mostly due to poor living conditions, living alone, financial strain, poor social support, lack of a care, poor contact with relatives and friends and poor physical health. As a result, overwhelming feelings of deprivation, loneliness and uselessness became common concerns (Department of Health, 2006).

Chi and Chou (2001) ascertain that social support from family is important for elderly Chinese people in Hong Kong. Other studies (Shetye, 2007) carried out in rural China indicated that the risk of depression for the elderly living in rural areas was lower than that in urban communities in China, and both were at a lower risk of depression than those in Western countries. The prevalence of Chinese tradition and culture may largely contribute to lower incidents of depression in urban areas of China.

In traditional Chinese families, it has been the norm for families to take care of the elderly, often living together in the same home; customarily three generations reside together. The current generation of the elderly in Hong Kong face new challenges as their children are now living and working abroad, or both husband and wife are working full time. Thus many of the elderly are now living alone or in elderly centres, further adding to feelings of isolation and separation from their core families. Lam and Boey (2005) claim that the Chinese community in Hong Kong used to consist of a closely knit family system that gave strong support for the elderly. Now this situation has changed, resulting in a high number of elderly living in old urban areas, a factor contributing to depression. To compound this matter, the elderly people are not vocal in expressing their needs and often stay away from seeking help from mental health professionals because of the fear of being stigmatized (Lam and Boey, 2005). The Life Garden Project played a part in helping the elderly with depressive symptoms to minimize depression, and helped them to express themselves and their needs in alternative ways to lessen the feeling of being stigmatized, art therapy being one of those interventions.

The art therapy groups of Life Garden

The project entailed three tiers of intervention. *Life Story Book Writing* aimed to help depressed elderly appreciate their life experiences and attainments. *Alternative Therapeutic Interventions* such as art therapy, music therapy and horticultural therapy helped to address emotional/psycho-social needs, as well as aromatherapy and auricular acupressure therapy to help with insomnia and ease depressive symptoms. *Home Spatial Design Work* provided the elderly with an opportunity to improve their home living environment (Evangelical Lutheran Church Social Service, 2009). The culmination of these approaches offered a holistic approach that aimed to improve the psychological wellbeing of elderly Life Garden clients in Hong Kong.

Aims

Art therapy, as part of the whole treatment plan for Life Garden, aimed to minimize features of depression for the elderly, enable them to express their thoughts and feelings using a non-verbal approach, build self-esteem, connect with others in a meaningful way, build a sense of belonging, and re-activate their potential in their day-to-day life. Features of depression include self-dislike, feelings of worthlessness, loss of gratification, loss of attachments, hopelessness, lethargy and guilt that manifest and are addressed in art therapy (Rubin, 1999; Wadeson, 1980). The Life Garden Art Therapy Groups offered a unique approach, blending Eastern ideologies by integrating Chinese traditions and value systems and incorporating a communal supportive approach with Western-based art therapy practice.

Overview of participants

The Life Garden Art Therapy Groups consisted of elderly men and women aged between 65 and 83 years old. Most of the clients were born and raised in mainland China and, due to the challenges of difficult living conditions in rural China and economic struggles, the majority have not had the opportunity to engage in art making in their lives. Most of the elderly were also not accustomed to verbalizing their issues/problems and sharing feelings, partly based upon cultural norms (Lo, 2004). Interaction with the art materials in art therapy gave the elderly an opportunity to touch their inner world in a less threatening way, and gave them a voice to say the things that words cannot always express.

Group format

There was one morning group and one afternoon group held each year for a total of three years. Each session was for two hours and met for ten consecutive weeks. I worked alongside the social worker on the team, who organized the details of the therapeutic groups. Although I could understand much of what was being said in Cantonese and could converse in simple Cantonese, one of the social worker's tasks was to translate when needed. After each group we would de-brief what had transpired in the group, taking note of the progress of each group member. If any issues came up for clients, we would contact Life Garden staff or case workers to support the client between the group meetings. Working as a part of a multidisciplinary team can enable the therapy work to extend out beyond the therapy room. Each session began with a verbal sharing time in which members shared their feelings about coming into the group and talked about their week or previous image.

We then came together to stretch and move to music as a warm-up exercise. Members were encouraged to create their own movement or dance as we moved through the circle. As the members became more comfortable with each other Tai Chi was also incorporated, where group members trained in Tai Chi led the exercise in a private outdoor space, moving and interacting with each other in a supportive way. Such movement exercises gave members an opportunity to connect. Tea time gave members time for social interaction. The rest of the session was dedicated to image making and then verbal sharing of their images within the group.

Week by week the members became more engaged in the art-making process and the sharing of their images within the group. More attention to the listening and sharing process gave members the opportunity to develop trust within the group and form group cohesion. The themes of the group in each session were designed to give the members an opportunity to use art as an expressive tool to explore their inner world, be in touch with feelings, explore their relationships in the past and in their current life, be in touch with memories, connect with others and find their own strengths.

Group process: 'Making art kitchen style'

Art-making time usually followed after sharing tea together sitting around the table. 'Making art kitchen style' is a rhetorical expression suggestive of an emphasis on the shared experience of creating art in the kitchen family style, echoing the process of cooking together in preparation for Chinese New Year, a time of togetherness in Chinese culture. Art materials were laid out in the middle of the table like ingredients being gathered for cooking and the group began to respond to the materials and soon to each other. Interacting with different art materials enabled the clients to begin to participate actively in making images, exercising the 'doing' aspect of art therapy. As stated by Rubin (1999), various art materials meet different needs of the client, and offering a variety gives the client choice to allow for personal expression.

In the first session the clients were invited to make an image to introduce themselves. Although a variety of materials were offered, clients tended to use magazines in the couple of sessions, as many of the elders did not have much experience in handling art materials and expressing themselves through images. But in the process of collecting pictures for their collage, clients began to collect pictures together, cutting out pictures of fruit and other food, and passing them around, gathering the ones that they connected with into their own pile. They created their collage like one would create a meal, while also being aware of the needs of others to complete their artwork by passing the glue and magazine pictures. Members provided assistance to each other until all images were complete. The process of sharing the artwork followed much like the above. At first the elderly needed some time to warm up to the process of sharing their images.

In the next session some of the members began to pick up drawing materials and began to draw. The group praised the ones that drew out their picture and encouraged others to also try to draw. By the fourth session members worked as partners to co-create an image using a combination of dry and wet materials. Most of them had moved away from using collage. By the fifth session, most members used a combination of oil pastels and paint to make their self-portrait. Having success with paint gave the clients confidence to try clay. The elderly responded well to the clay medium as they made clay containers connected to their family life, and plates to hold clay food, sharing stories of their happy and meaningful times with family during their childhood and for some shared meaningful memories with their life with their spouse.

As group trust developed, members were more able to express themselves through their pictures, and connect to a deeper personal meaning of what the pictures were saying. This was evident in the making and sharing of the self-portrait paintings. Through the sharing of this image most members walked away from the group with a higher sense of self-appreciation as they connected with positive attributes of themselves as reflected in the painting. Many members returned to the next session wanting to look at their painting again, and appeared more lively and engaged. By the end of the group, most members shared their images with the group with greater ease and deeper insight. They were able to express themselves and be heard and understood.

Research results

Participants of the Life Garden Art Therapy Groups were asked to complete the following assessments for assessing their emotional health before and after the programme: (1) Geriatric Depression Scale (GDS 15) (measuring levels of depressive symptoms); and (2) Kinetic House–Tree–Person (KHTP) projective drawing (indicators for overall functioning). Those who scored between 5 and 7 on the Geriatric Depression Scale indicated mild to moderate levels of depression.

Post-group participants scored an average of 1 to 3 on the Geriatric Depression Scale, indicating no to mild depressive symptoms. Comparing pre- and post-KHTP projective drawings, line qualities in the post drawings were generally more firm and interrupted, suggesting a more assertive and assured individual, and figures of the person were much larger, with more detail and colour, which may point towards a larger (bigger and stronger) sense of self-esteem, with more attention and detail to the self. This indicates a more connected state of self, more grounded or with more purpose (Burns, 1987).

Emerging themes in the Life Garden Art Therapy Groups

There were two main themes that emerged over the course of the art therapy groups which seemed to be related to community and traditional values.

Importance of community

Due to the overall lack of communal living and close connection to families and social support for today's elderly, the framework of the art therapy group was centred around creating a sense of community/communal living and social support, so that week by week the group became a safe haven for them to address their feelings about their life and what they had been through.

Overall, their connection with mainland China was deep. Many of the group members stated that 'China is great'; but in the same breath they also expressed times were tough living there as children, and there was no time to play. Most of them reported that they had never done art before and 'were no good'. So taking this into account, an emphasis on 'playing with' the art materials and engaging in the art-making process in art therapy helped them to find their voice within the context of honouring Chinese value systems and philosophy. Even though basic principles of the Western practice of art therapy were carried out, the driving force that led to the success of group cohesion was the integration of the group as a communal inner circle that echoed the sense of communal living they had lost in their lives.

According to Bond (1991) the advancement of closeness of an inner circle is based upon trust. Moreover, cross-cultural research on trust revealed that 'Chinese from the mainland and Hong Kong were more trusting towards this inner circle than were their comparable Americans' (p.37). For the group, creating an inner circle in which to share their memories, struggles and worries about their life was one way of building a sense of communal support. This inner circle developed out of paying tribute to customary traditions within the group process such as creating art in the kitchen family style (providing a kitchen-like atmosphere when making art), tea time (echoing the tea ceremony), moving/dancing/tai-chi together and sharing together around the table. The art therapy group was itself a container in which this inner circle could take shape; and I as the therapist held the process.

Figure 8.1 reflects the struggles that a client has endured and a search for life goals in his elder years. The green (bottom area) represents his need to seek a way out of his troubles throughout his life; the middle area corresponds to his efforts and hardship in his working career; and the top portion signifies his search to reach out and find his purpose in his elder years. Throughout the group process he experienced success in his ability to engage in art making, shared his life memories and difficulties and received recognition and praise from group members, which he had longed for in his life.

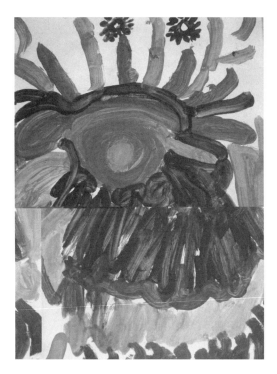

Figure 8.1 *Search for life goals*

A clay container (Figure 8.2) made by the same client holds his feelings of happiness and sadness. The camel and penguin represent his past hard life. The blue portion (dark area on right of rim) of the container symbolizes the dark side of the people in his life and the yellow and orange part (light area along the rim) the brightness. He expressed that he made connections with group members and realized that this connection had a positive impact upon his life.

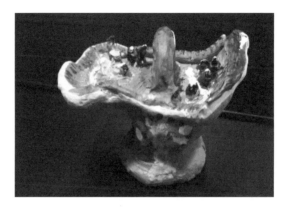

Figure 8.2 *Container of happiness and sadness*

The development of a communal inner circle comprised of sharing stories of the happy times they had as children, sharing in the customs and festivities of Chinese New Year with their parents, grandparents and relatives, making dumplings and tea time. For the elderly in the Life Garden Art Therapy Groups, these stories were by far the most treasured memories for most of them. As they had early rearing in the mainland, core Chinese cultural values and philosophy remained high and were still engrained for most of the elderly in the group. Figure 8.3 represents a client's happy feelings in her early days with her family during Chinese New Year. The dumplings represent reunion and the desire to have a family togetherness.

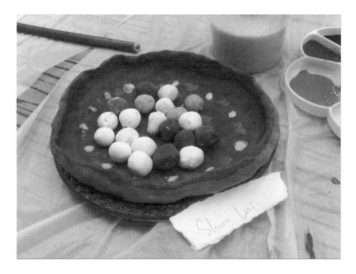

Figure 8.3 *Dumplings*

Chinese value systems

Traditional values linked to Chinese philosophy were ever present in the group, and paying tribute to them allowed the group to function most effectively in a natural way in respect to this paradigm, with filial piety, face and *Li* being the dominant ones emerging in the group. These concepts are described below.

Filial piety is acknowledged as the first virtue in Chinese culture. Rooted in Confucianism, the norm of *xiào* refers to deep loyalty to one's parents, and the norms of *rén and yì* (benevolence and righteousness) are extended to one's dealings with all elders (New World Encyclopedia, 2008). Filial piety is deeply engrained in Chinese culture, and for the group members it manifested on two levels: the elderly giving respect to their parents; and the children of the elderly carrying out filial responsibility to the elderly, their parents.

At times filial piety and face came together hand in hand; this was especially true at the second level. Some of the elderly would report that their sons or daughters 'were good, taking care of them so well and sending them money'. This can be seen as a kind of *face giving* statement to their adult children. Ananta and Arifin (2009) state that, as the norm of living together with elder parents has now changed, adult children carry out their filial piety through financial support or employing non-family caregivers.

Figure 8.4 represents this aspect of filial piety and a client giving face towards his mother. While making this image of his mother, he whispered to me that his mother was controlling, waving his arm while holding his paintbrush as if it were a stick. His eyes were big, yet he was smiling. But in the group sharing he described his mother as a 'good' and nice mother, always taking good care of him. (It was important to give respect to his mother in the group setting and mirror back to him the good nature of his mother that he had shared.) In the later phase of therapy the client brought up his mother again, voicing that she had done her best.

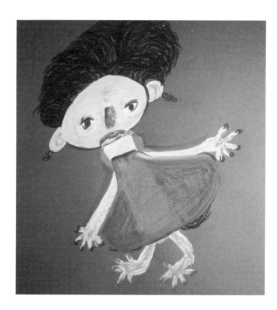

Figure 8.4 *Filial piety*

Li is a principle of Confucian ideas that is comprehensive. It embodies ceremonies, rituals or norms of proper social behaviour, with emphasis placed on social norms (Fung, 1966). Being attentive and sensitive to the needs of others is a significant component of *li*. It involves anticipating other people's needs and feelings without being told and responding to them (Gabrenya and Hwang, 1996). Group trust also developed out of the way group members exemplified *li* through their interactions with others in the group. *Li* helped members to build social support, as a majority of the group members who had a fair amount of mobility looked after the other less able-bodied ones like a 'third eye', not helping them too much, but extending their care and assistance. This *li* interaction seemed to become the group norm.

Conclusion

Art therapy, as part of the whole treatment plan for Life Garden, has been a successful means to enable the elderly to express their thoughts and feelings using a non-verbal approach. The interactions with the art materials gave the elderly an opportunity to touch their inner world in a less threatening way, and gave them a voice to say the things that words cannot always express.

As an alternative therapeutic approach, art therapy gives the elderly an opportunity to engage in the doing aspect of their life, as they need to do (make something) in art therapy. This 'doing' process enabled clients to 'do' and take action in their current life, helping them to invest or re-invest back into their life. At the end of the group, most members were visibly more interactive and engaged, and more enthusiastic about life. Art therapy enabled the elderly to tap into their own potentias and abilities in the elder years, and for most to activate their potential in their day-to-day life to find their place and personal value in this now modern Hong Kong society. By offering a communal living approach, important Chinese traditional values could be carried out and realized by creating an atmosphere of cohesiveness, support and sense of belonging within the group, echoing the importance of communal support in traditional Chinese community living.

Growing up in Hong Kong I have experienced Chinese cultural norms throughout my life; working here as an art therapist since 1995 has given me the opportunity to integrate these traditions into my work with clients and groups locally. The Life Garden Art Therapy Groups are one example of the importance of integrating group interconnection within the paradigm of core traditional values. It has been an honour to work with the elderly, and I thank them for all that they have shared.

References

Ananta, A. and Arifin, E. (2009) 'Older Persons in Southeast Asia: From Liability to Asset.' In: A. Ananta and E. Arifin (eds) *Older Persons in Southeast Asia: An Emerging Asset* (pp.3–46). Pasir Panjang, Singapore: Institute of Southeast Asian Studies.

Bond, M. (1991) *Beyond the Chinese Face: Insights from Psychology.* Hong Kong: Oxford University Press.

Burns, R. (1987) *Kinetic-House-Tree-Person Drawings (K-H-T-P): An Interpretative Manual.* New York, NY: Brunner/Mazel.

Census and Statistics Department (2006) *Hong Kong Census 2006.* Available at www.bycensus2006.gov.hk/FileManager/EN/Content_981/a103e.xls, accessed on 4 November 2011.

Census and Statistics Department (2011) *Hong Kong: The Facts.* Available at www.gov.hk/en/about/abouthk/factsheets/docs/population, accessed on 4 November 2011.

Chan, S.W.C., Chiu, H.F.K., Chien, W., Thompson, D.R. and Lam, L. (2006) 'Quality of life in Chinese elderly people with depression.' *International Journal of Geriatric Psychiatry 21,* 312–318.

Chi, I. and Chou, K. (2001) 'Social support and depression among elderly Chinese people in Hong Kong.' *International Journal of Aging and Human Development 52,* 3, 231–252.

Department of Health (2006) *Elderly Health Services Newsletter.* Available at www.info. gov.hk/elderly/english/healthinfo/healthproblems/depression.htm, accessed on 4 November 2011.

Evangelical Lutheran Church Social Service (2009) *Life Garden Manual.* Project Report. Hong Kong: Hong Kong Christian Social Service Department.

Fung, Y. (1966) *A Short History of Chinese Philosophy.* New York, NY: The Free Press.

Gabrenya, W. and Hwang, K. (1996) 'Chinese Social Interaction: Harmony and Hierarchy on the Good Earth.' In: M. Bond (ed.) *The Handbook of Chinese Psychology* (pp.36–54). New York, NY: Oxford University Press.

Lam, C.W. and Boey, K.W. (2005) 'The psychological well-being of the Chinese elderly living in old urban areas of Hong Kong: A social perspective.' *Aging and Mental Health 9,* 2, 162–166.

Lo, H.M. (2004) 'Social work intervention for people with depressive disorder.' *Hong Kong Practitioner 26,* 486–492.

New World Encyclopedia (2008) *Filial Piety.* Available at www.newworldencyclopedia. org/entry/Filial_piety, accessed on 4 November 2011.

Rubin, J. (1999) *Art Therapy: An Introduction.* Philadelphia, PA: Brunner/Mazel.

Shetye, S. (2007) *Prevalence and Correlates of Depression in Elderly Chinese in Hong Kong.* Masters thesis submitted for the Master of Public Health at the University of Hong Kong.

Wadeson, H. (1980) *Art Psychotherapy.* New York, NY: John Wiley & Sons.

Welsh, F. (1997) *A History of Hong Kong.* London, UK: HarperCollins.

PART 3

Integration of Spirituality

Chapter 9

New Consciousness on Art Therapy in Thailand Based on Spiritual Remedy

Anupan Pluckpankhajee

For thousands of years, people in Southeast Asia believed that they lived in a particular area called "*Suvarnabhumi*" or "Golden Land." Even though the origin of this word is unclear, its historical background can be traced back to the 2nd century bc. According to records, the great Buddhist patron, *King Asoka* of India, sent two Buddhist missionaries named *Sona Dhera* and *Uttara Dhera* to spread the word of Buddhism to distant areas, namely *Suvarnabhumi*. The notion of *Suvarnabhumi* appears in a number of historical accounts, for example as the "Golden Peninsula" in the legendary Hindu epic *Ramayana* (ancient scripture of India regarding religion and the culture of Brahmanism) and as the "Golden Island," one of the most civilized places on earth in *Ptolemy's*1 famous book *Geography* (Institute of Discovery and Creative Learning, 2007). Until today, the origin of *Suvarnabhumi* continues to be widely discussed amongst those in the ancient towns of Southeast Asia, from *Pakalanbujung* in Malaysia, to *Daruma* in Indonesia, *Wayatapura* in Cambodia, *Oc-eo* in Vietnam, and *Nakornpathom* in Thailand.

Suvarnabhumi: Where life developed with spiritual arts

Long before the establishment of the *Thai* people in *Suvarnabhumi*, Chinese and Indian civilizations had constantly expanded their influences

---

1   *Ptolemy* is the name Thai people use to call *Klaudios Ptolemaios* (85–168 ad; he was a geographer who had many famous academic works in the early Christian era).

over this area. Various artifacts from the "Iron Age" were excavated, all of which indicate that trade existed around 500 to 300 bc. In particular, ancient beads from the south of Thailand help to explain the continuous relationship between *Suvarnabhumi* and other civilizations in the world (Pongpanich, 2009).

The formation of Thai art identity began, coincidently, with the development of the nation-state between the 5th and 9th centuries. Different ideas were incorporated, which helped shape the traditional ways of living, such as the absolute monarchy; the *DunSun2* culture of ancient Mon; the *Sanskrit* language; Brahmanism; and Buddhism, witnessed in the existing cultural artifacts, religious sculptures, and Buddha images. This early process was closely involved with the concept of *Tantrayana* and the *Shiva* cults of *Brahmanism,3* both of which played essential roles in shaping the identity of Thai art (Krairoek, 2010).

Spiritual beliefs, Brahmanism, and Buddhism: The fundamental trinity

Spiritual beliefs, Brahmanism, and Buddhism laid a concrete foundation for the emergence of the *Suvarnabhumi* civilization. Such a civilization created certain forms of culture, customs, beliefs, art, therapy, and a prosperous lifestyle, as indicated in the ancient saying, "The water is full of fishes while the farm is full of rice." In Thailand's agricultural society, life relied heavily on spiritual concepts. There was a *soil spirit* (a mother of the land) for farming, a *rice spirit* (the goddess of rice) for food and wellbeing, and a *house spirit* for home protection. Brahmanism also influenced the pattern of politics, for instance the king was believed to be God's reincarnation, who held absolute power, and who resolved all suffering and maintained happiness amongst his people. The role of Brahmanism is further emphasized by the fact that the king's coronation is always conducted solely under Brahman concepts.

Medication or folk therapy was also influenced by Brahman beliefs. Accordingly, knowledge was delivered verbally, from one person to another. It was not until a later period that folk therapy was documented. Some doctors combined superstition in their treatment. These so-called

---

2   From the Chinese annals of the *Liang-shu* dynasty, *DunSun* meant five cities ruled by five kings. The cities were sited on a cape stretched out into the ocean. *DunSun* was one of the main commercial centers.

3   *Tantrayana* of Buddhism spread from India into *Suvarnabhumi* in the 8th century AD; *Shiva* of Hinduism spread to Cambodia during the middle of the 10th century AD.

"magical healings" are purported to be able to cure all illnesses with a mysterious magical power. Evidence of this healing appears in ancient verses, which can be interpreted as follows:

> One who wants to learn must choose a teacher with concern

> He should be eccentric knowing how to use magic

> Only being a teacher without a magical power

> Do not pick that type, people will be misguided.

According to the *History of Medication and Therapy*, an early manuscript on the healing process was discovered in the 8th century, during the reign of King *Singhanawat* of *Nanchao*. It was written in *Pali*, a language used in Buddhist *Tripitaka*. Hundreds of years later, in the 13th century, 102 buildings of *Arokaya Sala* (hospitals) were worshipfully constructed by the Great Cambodian King, *Jayavarman VII*. The setting up of *Arokaya Sala* represented the connection between religious beliefs and spiritual healing under the concept of *Mahayana* (a Buddhist instruction on how to concentrate in practice with industriousness to reach *Bodhisattva* to remove suffering). In addition to this, the *Mahayana* notion of *Bodhisattva* was highly revered as well as the image of *Bhaisajyaguru*, a specific posture in *Mahayana* Buddhism, believed to help cure all human diseases. As for *Theravada* Buddhism, certain forms of Buddhist artifacts were thought to be sacred remedies. They were put in water and prayed to by the patients, who later drank what they considered to be a special treatment.

However, an obvious relationship between Buddhism and medication can be seen in an ancient inscription, which was written in 1180. It explored the crucial motives behind King *Jayavarman VII*'s idea to build *Arokaya Sala*. The inscription reads, "Those who stand for me in the future, please keep in mind that…all merits I have made [building *Arokaya Sala*], should not be abandoned. Whoever maintains my wishes, will receive merits in return."

The disappearing of inner study

Over 100 years ago, modern education began in Thailand, as a consequence of Western influence. It then became a major goal for the country to reach world standards. Thus, modern education inspired the country to undergo rapid changes, both politically and socially. Prior to this change, knowledge of art, literature, warfare, medication, and therapy was only centered on the "temple" and the "palace," as mentioned in several ancient Thai inscriptions. With the expansion of modern education, traditional values such as local wisdom, religious cultures, and spiritual beliefs were greatly challenged by the so-called "scientific method" (Ngamvidhayapong, 2002). This new method replaced old values with the concepts of numbers, measurement, and empirical data. It did not take long to realize the impact of science, as it overturned traditional forms of learning and was developed into the mainstream Thai educational system. More importantly, once science stepped into the realms of art, therapy, and education, it deconstructed the perception of human beings. In doing so, the body, mind, and soul were now studied separately from each other. Prawase Wasi (2010), a well-acclaimed doctor and scholar, underlines this point by stating, "It [modern education] is based mainly on lessons and theories, but does not help one to understand oneself, not to mention our transformation" (p.32).

To understand further the differences between modern and traditional education, it's worth noting Sulak Sivaraksa's (2002) comments that from a Buddhist viewpoint education should be a process that allows people to discover their hidden abilities, understand themselves, and then help to create a peaceful society. According to the Buddhist perspective, knowledge can be divided into three categories: *Information*, a knowledge acquired from listening; *Rationalism*, a knowledge acquired from considering; and finally, *Pragmatism*, a knowledge acquired from practicing. The last category is known as *Sikkhā* or a common way of education, naturally practiced by all living beings to achieve their goals in life. In order to complete the learning, meditation, and the service mind, or the right thought (*Sammāsankappa*), the triumvirate of good manners, proper speech, and an uncorrupted career (*Silasikkhā*) are viewed as the keys to success. In brief, inner study, which has lost its significance over a period of time, is the process that raises self-awareness, social concern, and a sympathetic nature. Indeed, it is an education that takes life as a principle.

Art therapy: The rise of anthroposophy in Buddhist Thailand

From 1902, the public became familiar with the term "anthroposophy." This newly created term is derived from two Greek words, namely *Anthropos* and *Sophia*, which mean "man" and "wisdom." It was initiated by Dr. Rudolf Steiner (1865–1924), a German scholar and philosopher, whose study was in natural science, but who incorporated the philosophies of Goethe.4 Despite the fact that Steiner took an important role in theosophy in his early life, at the beginning of the 20th century he shifted his interests to anthroposophy. For Steiner, since 1914, anthroposophy is simply "spiritual science" (Steiner, 1991, p.66).

Core anthroposophic concept

In order to understand Steiner's concept, it is important to look at the contents of anthroposophy. The fundamental core of anthroposophy is to understand human beings through the three dimensions of Physical Body, Soul, and Spirit (Table 9.1). Furthermore, it talks about the concept of reincarnation, which is similar to Buddhist beliefs. Anthroposophy discusses various issues, such as the origin of birth, the way of living, causes of illness, and the correlation between the spiritual world and the actual world. According to this concept, human beings leave the spiritual world with a genuine wisdom, as a means to accomplish their mission in life. Once they die, they return to the spiritual world with greater wisdom. I will now explain the significance of these three dimensions.

Table 9.1 *Elements of life according to anthroposophy*

Body	Physical body Etheric body Astral body	Instinct Drive Desire
Soul	Sentient soul Intellectual soul Consciousness soul	Motive
Spirit	Spirit self Life spirit Spirit man	Wish Intent Decision

The Body Element

1. *Physical Body* is the organ of the body, which reacts simultaneously to changing situations. It is believed to center on four elements, namely Earth, Water, Air, and Fire. The Physical Body functions by "instinct."

---

4   *Johann Wolfgang Von Goethe* (1749–1832) was a German scientist, philosopher, and writer who was top in his field, whether it was science or art.

2. *Etheric Body* concerns the energy that makes the body grow. It is common to humans, animals, and plants. The Etheric Body functions by "drive."

3. *Astral Body* deals with feelings. It is common to humans and animals. The Astral Body functions by "desire."

The Soul Element

1. *Sentient Soul* is the soul that perceives the outside world through the astral body, which then causes desire and feelings, such as anger, love, and sorrow, to take place in the soul. It is common to both humans and animals and it functions by "motive.'

2. *Intellectual Soul* is one higher than the sentient soul; it is directed by rationality but still connects to the sentient soul, and also functions by "motive."

3. *Consciousness Soul* is the deep consciousness inside the soul, without any prejudice at all, and it also functions by "motive."

The Spirit Element

1. *Spirit Self* is the spirit of each person that perceives the spiritual world through the enlightenment that flashes inside oneself. It is the result of feelings, reflected when one perceives the physical world.

2. *Life Spirit* is the life power of the developed spirit that works on intention.

3. *Spirit Man* is the person whose soul is free from the physical world. His spiritual world was already developed.

Connection to art therapy

At the beginning of the 20th century, "spiritual science" became a major force in broadening the knowledge of medication, art therapy, architecture, bio-dynamic agriculture, conventional study, and alternative study on a much wider scale (Lissau, 2008). Steiner's work on anthroposophical art therapy required a basic knowledge in anthroposophy as well as the arts, with the supporting skills of spiritual comprehension, medication, and therapy. These are the reasons why art therapy is different from conventional medicine. Art therapy has a unique procedure for diagnosing symptoms, which involves coloring, shading, painting, drawing, forming, and making shapes. All of these elements are also viewed as methods of treatment in the process of art therapy.

Art is thoughtfully implemented during the therapy process. In doing so, the whole process can be seen as aesthetic, similar to Buddhist ideas recorded by *Buddhadasa Bhikkhu* that art is beauty and is the result of practice (Buddhadasa Bhikkhu, 2006). In this sense, anthroposophical art therapy emphasizes the beauty of the procedure and its outcome. In other words, it can simply be stated that therapy is art.

Spiritual aspects of anthroposophical art therapy

As mentioned previously, anthroposophical medicine is focused on the balance between being healthy and being ill. Therefore, the aim of anthroposophical medicine is not just to cure the illness, but also to balance the dynamics in the human body (Table 9.2). There are several techniques of art therapy, which offer a series of suitable therapeutic methods for each of the various symptoms from which unbalanced qualities appear in the artworks. This chapter will focus on painting and line drawing in particular.

Table 9.2 *The relationship between body, soul, and spirit, and the process of anthroposophic art therapy*

Head	Drawing	Light & dark Dynamic Form Rhythm	I Thinking (nervous system) **Astral**
Heart	Painting	Close & open Warm & cool Silence & social	Feeling (rhythmic system) **Etheric**
Hand	Clay	Logic Movement Lively	Willing (metabolic system) **Physical Body**

There is one German word which is interesting to look at, namely *Organpsyche*. It can be interpreted as "every organ relates to spirit." As such, art therapy shares the same view with modern medicine, that illness can be examined through the function of organs. In fact, anthroposophy focuses specifically on the liver, kidney, heart, and lungs as being the cause of human illness (Kutsch, 2005).

Anthroposophical art therapy considers art as taking both forms of outward expression and internal feeling. Thus, treatment by art therapy is practiced from outside to cure the illness inside, to create inner balance, or to release the tensions from within. Art is not just a method; it is a genuine medicine that helps people to regain a balanced life. I will now further describe the important quality of art therapy techniques such as coloring and line drawing.

COLOR

This world is full of colors, for instance the clear *blue* sky, the *emerald green* sea, the *deep blue* mountain, the blooming *yellowish* flowers. It is the sunlight that makes colors visible to humans, who later realize the different quality of each color. The core concept of anthroposophy mainly relies on two color theories, one created in 1791 by Goethe (1976) and the other in 1921 by Steiner (1973). These theories clearly indicate that colors have an effect on the development of a human's inner senses. The interaction between them is that, whilst humans are influenced by looking at colors, colors are also used by humans to express their inner feelings.

1. *Blue* is a powerful color. Yet, it signifies silence, coldness, sorrow, and embrace.

2. *Yellow* represents the sun. Its center is strong and intensive, gradually becoming lighter at the edge.

3. *Red* is an active color. It provokes awareness, stimulation, and hotness.

4. *Green* is the combination of yellow and blue colors. It implies a self-balancing quality. Therefore, to look at the green environment, when feeling tired, will help to refresh.

5. *Orange* is based on yellow and red; its combination can be seen as a fusion of light and heat, suggesting an awakening character.

6. *Purple* is a mixture of blue and red. This color has a special feature, which can relate to the human mind. Whilst the lighter purple provides a feeling of comfort, the deep purple invokes a feeling of mystery.

These above explanations can be summed up in Goethe's beliefs, as color not only affects external relations, but internal ones as well. The quality and awareness of color appears in the painter's mind.

Form

Humans and plants share a mutual connection. Their forms are created by lines and curves, which are influenced by the impressions of the world and the universe. Whilst the curve is believed to come from the cosmic power, the line is made by the world power. Each form has a different implication, for example the triangle represents universal power, and the square represents the earth's power. When a child, aged between four and seven years old, draws a house by combining the triangle with the square, it relates to a "triangular roof," which signifies a protective feeling, whilst the square wall symbolizes a secure feeling. Everything surrounding us has a different figure and form, which has an impact on the human mind. This world generates specific pictures for us. When a person starts drawing and coloring a picture, it is, in fact, a mirror that is reflecting what is in their mind. Accordingly, it is not surprising that children begin their first drawing with a circle, triangle, and square; it is a result of what they perceive.

Line

For art therapy, a line is important for both functions of expression and impression. It relates to the physical body, attitudes, and emotions. Patterns of lines vary between straight, horizontal, free-form, diagonal, and curved. Once these skills are practiced in art therapy, they are called "form drawing" techniques, which are seen as one of the important therapies besides painting.

Buddhism and anthroposophic art therapy

There is one question that needs to be answered. How can anthroposophical art therapy have room to grow in Thailand, a country where Buddhism has successfully prevailed for centuries? The answer is because *Buddhism and anthroposophical art therapy are not the same and yet not different*. In this sense, art therapy falls into the Buddhist doctrine of "*Margga*" or "approach." The Buddhist religion does not guide followers to believe, but rather to practice and realize the consequence by themselves. Similarly, art therapy improves the patient's physical body, soul, and spirit through art making, which mirrors Buddhist meditation, and aims to raise awareness in the ever-changing state of the mind.

In 2004, two decades after Dr. Michaela Glöckler (Head of the Anthroposophy Medical Department at Goetheanum, Switzerland) gave an important speech to Thai scholars, art therapy in Thailand began to take a clear shape. At this time *Samitivej Srinakarin* Hospital launched a new section of Anthroposophical Art Therapy, which became a successful case study, largely followed by both government and private sectors. It cannot be denied that the growth of art therapy in Thailand is related to the widespread alternative education in the country. Within ten years, the popularity of art therapy was seen increasingly in schools, operating inside and outside Bangkok, and in anthroposophic networks, supported by art therapy organizations, such as *Therapeutikum am Kräherwald* and *Siebenzwerge* from Germany and *Zentrum zur Forderung anthroposophischer Kunsttherapie und Padagogik* in Thailand.

Case study: 53-year-old woman

To demonstrate these ideas, I will refer to my work with a 53-year-old woman. She is pale, slightly plump, and has straight short hair, with deep wrinkles on her forehead and tiredness in her eyes. She has struggled with depression for nearly 20 years, receiving treatment in Thailand as well as abroad. Throughout art therapy, she also took medication.

At first, she seemed to question how much art therapy would help. Her anxiety could be seen in her repeated questions. The first three sessions of art therapy introduced her to "free painting", "free drawing," and "free clay." These three methods have two essential targets. First, these procedures led the art therapist to understand the woman's "microcosmos" (Body, Soul, and Spirit), whether in balance or disrupted. Generally speaking, the body element (Physical, Etheric, and Astral) of art creations from the therapy session can be observed through the appearance of the painting, drawing, and clay, without the purpose of identifying "what it is." Rather, the art therapy process examines art in terms of the objective, for example the elements of colors and lines; are they hot, cold, heavy, light, pale, spreading, limited, sharp, moving, or static? Also, it focuses on how the patient expresses through art because it is closely associated with illness, spirits, and Steiner's categorization of temperament as either melancholic, choleric, phlegmatic, or sanguine. The second essential target is the spiritual relationship between the art therapist and the patient, which is explained in Table 9.3.

Table 9.3 *Spiritual relationship with client*

Therapist	Patient	
I (Ego) ⟶	Astral	If the patient has problems with the Astral Body, the therapist will work with the I.
Astral ⟶	Etheric	If the patient has problems with the Etheric Body, the therapist will work with the Astral.
Etheric ⟶	Physical Body	If the patient has problems with the Physical Body, the therapist will work with the Etheric.

An analysis of art therapy as a healing method

Looking at the patient's method of "free painting," her picture showed that all the colors were in stripes, detached from one another. It signified introversion and weakness, in response to her original disbeliefs in the art therapy process. A feeling of hopelessness overcame her. In anthroposophic terms, her Etheric Body confirmed she had a psychiatric problem. Her sickness related to the liver function, which represented the water element affecting her life.

The suitable method of therapy

For this patient, the suitable method was to harmonize the relationship from inside (introvert) to outside (extrovert). In doing so, the therapy focused on using activating colors and dynamic consciousness to make the patient capable of expressing her frustrations. Accordingly, the charcoal technique was the best choice to apply, because it emphasized line movement. The art therapist suggested that the patient look at the Italian Renaissance painter Rafael's work and duplicate it (Mees-Christeller, 1996). This method is very new in Thailand and it is not widely known amongst the Thai patients. Therefore, I chose to closely follow this established anthroposophic technique of copying the work of Rafael because of his use of line. Unlike familiar traditional Thai images, Rafael's images do not stir Thai people's feelings or memories, which would distract them from the healing process. More importantly, a group of anthroposophic art therapists claimed that the inner senses would be improved by copying the work of Rafael. I also assigned the patient to create watercolor paintings using four different shades, corresponding to different times of the day: morning, afternoon, evening, and night.

The result of art therapy

The 36 sessions undertaken by this patient lasted for more than a year. The results can be seen in the patient herself. She became joyful, livelier, and more focused. She had a new attitude following her experience in art therapy; she truly believed that art could resolve her inner problems. As a consequence of the therapy, this woman acquired an ability to calm herself when she began to feel depressed or aroused. She seemed to develop the capacity to be more flexible and less controlling. In addition, she began to realize that compromising made her life more attractive and pleasurable.

Conclusion

It is unfortunate that modern Thai education only emphasizes how to acknowledge the observable world, a complete change from the traditional one that focused on one's inner self. This misdirection has contributed to the present upheavals, existing at both the individual and the social level. Whether the anthroposophic ideal of a "balancing act" and Buddhist *Nirvāna* share the same concept or not, the growing popularity of anthroposophy in Thailand indicates that there is a common consciousness in this universe.

References

Bhikkhu, B. (2006) *Silapa Hang Kwarm Suk* [Art of Happiness]. Bangkok, Thailand: Sookaphapjai Publishing.

Goethe, J.W. (1976) *Theory of Colors*. Cambridge, MA: MIT Press.

Institute of Discovery and Creative Learning (2007) *The Account of Thailand*. Bangkok, Thailand: Institute of Discovery and Creative Learning.

Krairoek, P. (2010) *Rak Ngow Hang Silapa Thai* [Origins of Thai Art]. Bangkok, Thailand: River Books.

Kutsch, B. (2005) *Künsterische Therapie in der Fortbildung* [Advanced Artistic Therapy: Lecture Notes]. Bad Boll, Germany: Margarethe Hauschka-Schule.

Lissau, R. (2008) *Rudolf Steiner: A Teacher from the West* [Trans. Raveemas Promsiri]. Bangkok, Thailand: Suan Ngern Mee Ma Publishing.

Mees-Christeller, E. (1996) *Heilende Kunst und Künstlerisches Heilen* [Healing Arts and Artistic Healing]. Dornach, Switzerland: Futurum.

Ngamvidhayapong, O. (2002) *Patiroop Karn Suksa Moommong Tang Krabuanthat Lae Boribot Sungkom Thai* [The Reformation of Education from a Thai Perspective]. Chiangmai, Thailand: Midnight University. Available at http://61.47.2.69/~midnight/midculture44/newpage4.html, accessed on 28 January 2011.

Pongpanich, B. (2009) *Beyond Beads*. Bangkok, Thailand: Matichon Press.

Sivaraksa, S. (2002) *Karn Suksa Thai Tang Luerk Nai Anakot* [Thai Education: Future Alternative]. Available at www.sulak-sivaraksa.org/th/index.php?option=com_con tent&task=view&id=348&Itemis=44, accessed on 21 January 2011.

Steiner, R. (1973) *Das Wesen der Farben* [Color Theory]. Dornach, Switzerland: Rudolf Steiner Verlag.

Steiner, R. (1991) *Human and Cosmic Thought*. Stuttgart, Germany: Rudolf Steiner Press.

Wasi, P. (2010) *Thamachart Khong Supasing: Karn Khaothung Kwarm Jring Tangmod* [Nature of Everything: Access to Whole Truth]. Bangkok, Thailand: Green Panyayan Publishing.

Chapter 10

Art Therapy Inspired by Buddhism

Yen Chua

As an artist and art therapist practising in Asia with a Western fine arts training, Chinese Taoist roots and Vajrayana Buddhist faith, I see immense opportunities for developing new and meaningful intervention models. It is my own personal experience with art, art therapy and healing over the last two decades which leads me to believe that such a union is possible, desirable and beneficial. Over the past three years, I have tried to develop several intervention models for my Buddhist and non-Buddhist clients which are inspired by my immediate cultural and spiritual heritage, specifically Buddhism.

Although there is growing homogeneity between the East and the West due to globalization, the need to make significant adjustments to account for Asian sensibility, sensitivity, culture, lifestyle and religion, which divide these two worlds, remains unchanged. When I call for art therapy with an Asian flavour, I have two main reasons. First, because there is a great difference between the East and the West when it comes to culture and tradition and, second, because the East has much to offer and inform art therapy practice. I feel strongly that if we do not share our Asian history and traditions it would be a great loss and disservice to the global art therapy theory, practice and profession.

It is self-evident that, for art therapy to work, the art therapist needs to understand and appreciate the cultural and social background of his or her client. His or her efficacy as an art therapist and ability to benefit the client is very much dependent on his or her knowledge and understanding of the environment of his or her practice. When we talk about perceptions, relationships and patterns of interactions with our environment, it is inevitable that social and cultural conditionings play a very important role. Since these factors have a major influence on how clients perceive, relate and interact with their environment, it is important that art therapists are able to appreciate and understand these culture and value systems.

Revisiting art therapy in a Buddhist context: Considerations of the perceived dichotomy between science and spirituality

The worlds of psychology and religion have always been looked upon as two entirely different and perhaps incompatible realms, but when it comes to art therapy, this may not be the case. Both psychology and religion use the symbolic and transformative power of art to achieve their goals. In medical terminology, symbols reveal mental health, while in spiritual terminology they are used to cultivate happiness and peace of mind. In Buddhism and Hinduism, the transformative and healing power of art has always been appreciated and utilized to achieve the aforementioned purpose. They, just like art therapists, have not only tapped the power of art itself, but have also used the art-making process for such purposes for more than two millennia.

As a practising Buddhist familiar with different rituals and mind-training exercises employed to achieve self-awareness, understanding and peace of mind, I see great potential for the use and adaptation of the principles behind these practices in the development of culturally relevant art therapy intervention models. This observation is not new. In fact, during the early stages of modern psychology, Western psychologists were interested in this same idea. According to Katz (as cited in Norbu, 1992), 'Carl Jung was perhaps the first Western psychologist to be interested in Buddhism' (p.26). He was greatly interested in the use of symbolism in Buddhism, specifically the mandala and the intricate visualization practices associated with it. In this regards, Jung (1989) wrote, 'I knew that in finding the mandala as an expression of the self I had attained what was for me the ultimate' (p.197). Perhaps what drew Jung and many other students of psychology towards Buddhism is the fact that Buddhist texts and practices contain extensive exploration and detailed explanation about the working of the human mind and its nature.

Chogyam Trungpa Rinpoche once famously said that Buddhism will come to the West as a psychology (Fischer, 2004). According to Dzogchen Ponlop Rinpoche (1992), a renowned Buddhist master, 'Buddhist spiritual teachings present a genuine science of mind that allows one to uncover this inner reality, the nature of the mind and the phenomena that our mind experiences' (p.1). Further, His Holiness the Dalai Lama (2003) wrote that 'Buddhism, an ancient Indian thought, reflects a deep investigation into the workings of the mind' (para.6). This knowledge gained from more than 2000 years of study and experimentation with the human mind, and the repositories of artworks and art creation techniques of this spiritual tradition, can be a literal treasure trove, which has not even been scraped at the surface. The rituals, practices and processes these traditions employed can be a rich resource and template for modern art therapists to study, understand and if possible adapt to use, with more scientifically and proven theories as support. Meditation is another area where I believe a lot can be achieved. According to McNiff (1998), 'The practice of sitting meditation can be integrated with reflection on artistic images' (p.186).

Although introducing new therapeutic interventions inspired by knowledge and wisdom from our ancient religious and spiritual traditions may sound very unscientific, when it comes to art therapy and Buddhism a very logical and convincing case can be made. The fact that Buddhism also stresses a scientific approach of inquiry and verification helps greatly. In fact, Buddha's own advice to knowledge and wisdom disciples was 'Just as a goldsmith would test his gold by burning, cutting, and rubbing it, so you must examine my words and accept them, but not merely out of reverence for me' (Dalai Lama, 1995, p.26). The practitioners who used the meditations, visualization techniques and rituals studied the teachings on which they were based and have tried and tested them for centuries. It was this very idea of promoting cooperation between science and spirituality that inspired Chilean biologist, philosopher and neuroscientist Francisco Javier Varela García to found the Mind and Life Institute (MLI). Multi-disciplinary investigations and research in the traditional mind sciences, social sciences, contemplative scholarship and practice, philosophy and humanities are being conducted by MLI 'with the conviction that such collaboration could potentially be very beneficial to both modern science and to humanity in general' (MLI, n.d., para.8).

Over the last 15 years the psychology field has seen a resurgence in the use of mindfulness for a variety of conditions. According to Fields (2009), 'Buddhism and mindfulness is capturing the interest, heart, and imagination of the counseling field' (para.1). Meditation and mindfulness practices are being used effectively for the treatment of stress, anxiety, depression, pain and personality disorders. According to Watson (2001), 'Buddhism's centuries of exploration of subjective mind states may be a resource for Western science' (para.8). In fact, many of these rituals, artworks and art creation processes (whether physical or mental such as visualization of mandalas) are used very effectively to achieve desired mental or spiritual states. I think these techniques can and should be explored and adapted by art therapists today. In some sense, these people who formulated these elaborate techniques are the pioneers of our tradition.

As an artist, Buddhist and practising art therapist, I see great potential in this area because, in my own personal journey of healing and self-discovery, both my profession as an artist and spiritual practice played very important and harmonious roles. This experience gave birth to two important realizations. First, that art in itself, if used as a medium of exploring and understanding self-identity and nature, has great revelatory and healing power. Second, these spiritual traditions which have a history of using art to aid such contemplation, examination and reflection can also contribute greatly to this journey of healing and self-discovery and should not be shunned as unscientific or antiquated. Having made these two observations, I would like to share two intervention models from the many that I have developed based on these ideas. The first one was designed for my general clients, but inspired by certain Buddhist wisdom, practices and rituals. The second was designed for my Buddhist clients and inspired by different art therapy intervention models that I have come across and ideas I have myself come up with while teaching art for almost a decade and a half.

Art therapy inspired by Buddhist wisdom, practices and rituals

Although this intervention model is inspired by Buddhist wisdom, practices and rituals, the aim was to secularize these ideas and techniques to help my non-Buddhist clients develop emotional and mental wellbeing. As a result, these interventions can be used for clients who may not necessarily be Buddhist.

Being in the 'here and now'

According to Kabat-Zinn (2005), 'Mindfulness is a systematic approach to developing new kinds of control and wisdom in our lives' (p.2). While I do not specifically instruct my non-Buddhist clients to meditate before they begin making art, I consider it very important and always make an effort to allow them to settle down, calm their mind and be peaceful for a while, so that they are fully engaged and aware during the entire art-making process. Siegel (2007) wrote, 'Being aware of the fullness of our experience awakens us to the inner world of our mind' (p.3). Usually we are so caught up in what we are thinking and doing that we are tense and unaware of what is really happening around us. This lack of awareness numbs us and decreases the impact of the therapy process on us. A brief moment of meditative repose, mindful silence and relaxation can help calm the mind, settle in the present moment and concentrate on the task at hand. Such moments can bring clarity of thought and purpose, which is very beneficial for art making and art therapy. In addition to more purposeful art experiences, mindfulness can 'improve the capacity to regulate emotion, to combat emotional dysfunction, to improve patterns of thinking, and to reduce negative mindsets' (Siegel, 2007, p.5).

When I begin my session, I ask my clients to be attentive to the present moment, often referred to as the 'here and now'. I ask them to sit silently for a brief period and be calm. Asking the clients to take a short meditative break before starting the session is possible without affecting or offending their religious sensitivities, because some form of meditative reflection is practised in most global religious traditions. Meditation is simply being mindful and aware. Even in a secular setting, it is a recommended practice for anyone who would like to cultivate a sense of peace and calmness. Although there are many different spiritual and secular ways of achieving this calm, it can be achieved by giving a few simple instructions like, 'Take a few deep breaths, put everything aside, bring yourself to this room, be here and now, be present in the moment and relax…etc.'

After the art-making process and before the sharing begins, I also try to allow a pause and give time for settling down and reflection. I find that, for a meaningful sharing to occur, proper reflection on the part of the client needs to take place. Meditation masters have often used the metaphor of a calm lake, which is necessary for the best reflection of the sky, to stress that, to be aware of how our minds work and how our emotions control and drive us, we need to have calm and clear minds. The purpose of this contemplation break after the art-making session is to allow all raw emotions and disturbed thoughts that arose during the art-making session to settle. It also gives the clients time to compose their thoughts and look at whatever happened during the art-making process in a more objective and profound way.

Envisioning a 'perfect self'

Vajrayana or Tantric Buddhism employs deity visualization techniques during which the practitioner focuses on and identifies with the qualities of certain aspirational *Yidams* (meditation deities), like *Mañjuśrī*, the Buddha of Transcendental Wisdom, and *Avalokiteśvara*, the Buddha of Compassion. Yidams are the immaculate reflection or representation of the primordial and innate true nature of our own mind. In layman's language, they are the representation of us in our perfect form. What Buddha taught, in his Vajrayana teachings, is that in reality all of us are perfect. The Yidam visualization is therefore a powerful technique which has been used for centuries to acquaint or reacquaint practitioners with their true nature and hidden potential. According to Beer (2004), 'Deity Yoga employs highly refined techniques of creative imagination, visualization, and photism in order to self-identify with the divine form and qualities of a particular deity as the union of method or skillful means and wisdom' (p.142). When Vajrayana practitioners visualize the images or the form of a Yidam with its specific qualities, it is to help them work with their own mind to realize their own true nature.

To assist in this process, we can derive inspiration from the Buddhist concept of ten negative and ten positive deeds or actions. The ten negative deeds are very much like the 'thou shall not' of the Ten Commandments and the ten positive deeds are the 'thou shall' ones. Decreasing the former and increasing the latter is taught as the path to enlightenment or achievement of perfection. This teaching runs parallel to the common sense that committing fewer mistakes and doing more good deeds will lead to a happier and better self. This idea can be incorporated to help clients minimize their shortcomings and weaknesses and maximize their positive attributes or acquiring positive traits that lead to self-improvement and perfection.

While the Yidam visualization technique itself is complicated and is an esoteric practice that needs guidance and permission, there are core elements that I can use in my practice without contravening these codes. Some of the principles behind this technique are instructive and effective and therefore can be used to inspire someone to envision true potential and work towards this goal. I developed the intervention 'My Perfect Self' to help my clients visualize and work towards a better self.

Clients are first asked to envision or visualize themselves in perfect form with all aspirational qualities realized. After the visualization, they create a representational drawing of that perfect self. As Buddhist practitioners realized long ago, seeing the representation of an actualization potential or dream can be a very powerful motivating force. Seeing what is possible motivates people to work harder and realize their dreams. When making this representation, the client is asked to think of and then use various symbols to signify the desired attributes of this perfect self.

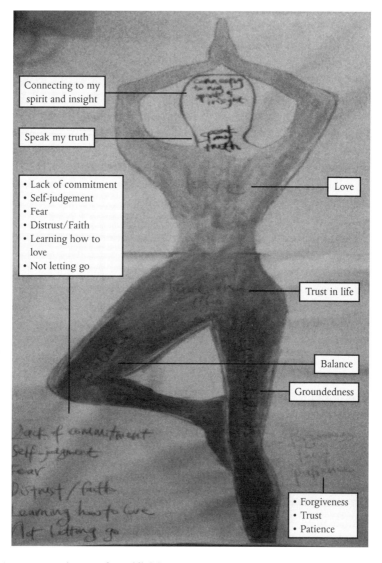

Figure 10.1 *'My Perfect Self' (1)*

Following this step, clients are then asked to either draw or list on the left side of the perfect self picture, using symbols or words, a few important deficiencies or negative qualities which are preventing them from realizing this perfect self. Next, on the right side, they draw or list certain qualities, which they require or may already possess, but need to amplify or improve upon, to realize the perfect self. Figures 10.1 and 10.2 are examples of 'My Perfect Self'. In order to make their writing more legible, I have added annotations to these photographs.

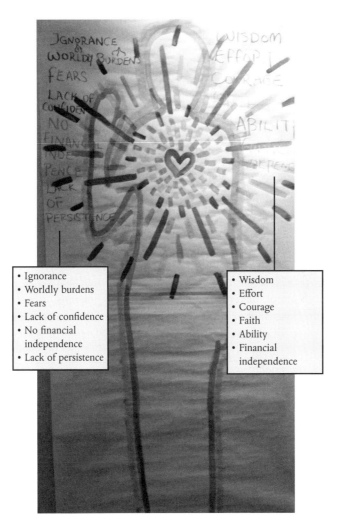

Figure 10.2 *'My Perfect Self' (2)*

Art therapy intervention for Buddhist clients

As previously stated, Tantric or esoteric Buddhism has used art and the art creation process for various purposes like meditation to achieve focus and concentration and as a medium to introduce and illustrate concepts like impermanence and interdependence through symbolic metaphors. Inspired by the idea of integrating my art therapy background with my knowledge of Buddhism, I started a group to help my Buddhist clients gain a clearer understanding of core Buddhist teachings and values, and thus promote spiritual wellbeing.

Over eight to ten sessions, I explored with the group members important Buddhist concepts like attachment, aversion, compassion, self-perception, suffering, happiness, interdependence, rebirth, the law of Karma, virtue and wisdom. At the beginning of each session, after going through the usual preparation routine, I asked the group to think about a specific Buddhist principle to use for art making. I based the media on the nature of the concept I wanted them to explore on that particular day. During these workshops, the participants not only gained greater clarity and understanding of important Buddhist ideas, but also appreciated how the teachings were relevant and applicable to their own lives, as well as the lives of their fellow participants. The sharing sessions which followed each episode of art making also allowed them to compare their interpretations and, at times, clarify their understanding of these principles.

While working on the concept of aversion or hatred, I used my knowledge about materials and asked the participants to use clay to create an object that represented what they thought was their enemy. After a group-sharing session on the nature of aversion or hatred from a Buddhist and Buddhist practitioner's perspective, I encouraged them to transform the enemy into something else based on the realization they gained during the art-making process and sharing session. Surprisingly, many participants were able to transform the enemy into something more positive or friendly.

During some of the sessions, certain concepts like 'attachment and aversion', 'suffering and happiness' and 'compassion and wisdom' were deliberately paired so that the participants could appreciate these concepts in a more comprehensive manner. The purpose was to help them experience the underlying dichotomous, but also complementary, relationship, which is a very important realization a Buddhist practitioner must make. I asked the participants to divide the paper into two or three folds and draw their interpretation of one concept on each side so that their juxtaposition would allow for a comparison and contrast to aid further exploration of the relationships. Through this process a client expressed her realization of the Buddhist concept that compassion and wisdom go hand in hand.

I used the same technique to address the concept of reincarnation and cyclic existence. The participants were asked to fold their art paper into three parts with each panel serving as a canvas for each phase of their life: the past, the present and the future. When we explored the purpose of the dedication of merits (acts to elevate spirituality), the participants actually created an artwork which could be offered as a dedication.

In addition to exploring specific Buddhist concepts, I also facilitated groups that allowed the participants to reflect on how their lives reflect Buddhist ideals. To achieve this goal, I developed an intervention called 'Action and Result'. Each participant in the group was provided with a sheet of paper and asked to depict on one half of the paper an action (positive or negative) that they performed in the past. On the other half, they were asked to depict the consequences of that action which they have experienced or are still experiencing at present. After the art making was complete, the participants were asked to reflect upon the relationship between their actions and its consequences in their present lives. This practice is a 'Buddhist After-Action Review'. The participants were encouraged to reflect upon how their actions had profound consequences on their lives and why it was important to be mindful about each of their actions. We reflected on how, once it was performed, they then had to bear the consequences of these actions, whether positive or negative.

My purpose behind developing this exercise was to help the participants reflect upon the relationship between their actions and its consequences. The Law of Karma, an important Buddhist tenet, teaches that each and every action (Karma) has its reciprocal result (Phala). Although most Buddhists know this concept and accept it to be true (because without accepting it, one cannot really be a Buddhist), often it remains just an idea or concept in mind. Many never really sit down and perform any introspection on how profound the principle itself is and the various implications it has in their lives. This intervention provided a time and space for participants to review and reflect upon their own actions and resulting consequences. This exercise has proven itself to be a powerful way to drive home the real understanding of the teaching of the Law of Karma.

Subsequent group sharing after the personal reflection segment illustrated that this helped develop an appreciation of the principle on a very personal level and brought its relevance and truth to light for the participants. It was no longer an abstract theory or principle but something they found to be real in their own lives. For example, Figure 10.3 was created by a participant whose relative had passed on because of a terminal disease. This intervention provided her with the opportunity to understand and process the emotional burden she carried and understand the profundity of her actions on her life. The participant realized that she was living with feelings of guilt, because she felt that she had taken her loved one for granted, and now wished that she had paid more attention to the relative when she was alive.

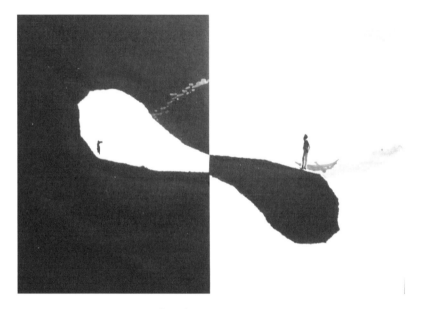

Figure 10.3 *Compassion and wisdom*

Discussion

Art therapy is an evolving practice, and I believe that it is incumbent upon us to enrich this practice by sharing with others our personal experiences and creating newer and more meaningful intervention models with the ultimate aim of benefiting our clients. During my study and practice, at times I encountered strict dogmatism and rigid interpretations of art therapy concepts, such as ideas on therapeutic boundaries. I believe that the journey of self-discovery and self-realization is very personal, intimate and unique in nature. Our best contribution can be sharing our own experiences and observations in the hope that they can benefit a fellow traveller. This idea is rooted in my Buddhist belief, as in Buddhism there is no concept of an intervening saviour. Buddha is seen as a benevolent friend who guides us on the path to enlightenment. The journey always has to be our own. Being a Buddhist and an art therapist whose ultimate aim is to benefit my clients in whichever way I can, I have learnt to look beyond these concepts and ideology to focus on the main intention behind them and never lose sight of my raison d'être as an art therapist. This motivation inspires me to learn more, work harder and come up with new intervention models inspired by my cultural context.

When I design my workshops, for example my Buddhist art therapy workshops, my purpose and intention is never to preach my interpretation of Buddha's teachings to my clients but rather to help them explore, clarify, compare and reflect on these important concepts on their own and as a result gain a more profound understanding about the meaning and implications of these teachings. I see the art creation process as a method, the art therapist as a facilitator and guide, and group members as fellow companions on the path of self-discovery and enlightenment. This model has great resonance with the Buddhist idea of Triple Gems: Buddha as the guide, Dharma (teaching) as the path and the Sangha (community) as the companion. Amazingly, this idea of companionship seems to resonate in the participants too. It is to their credit that several months after the first workshop they still find time to meet up once in a while and maintain the sense of communion and fellowship that was established during the workshop.

My approach is the same when I work with my non-Buddhist clients too. I believe that self-realization is much more meaningful and powerful than external intervention. Therefore, I see my role as an art therapist as primarily to provide a framework in which therapy can occur. The journey is, and should always be, the clients'. Unless my intervention becomes absolutely necessary, I usually limit my role to that of a facilitator, friend and companion who has been on the journey before or knows the path well and can therefore provide some helpful tips whenever needed.

Conclusion

I have been an artist for about two decades and have taught art and have been a Buddhist for more than a decade and a half. Over the last five years, two years of training and three of practice, I have had the good fortune to work as an art therapist in many settings, including a hospital, prison, youth care and rehabilitation, wellness centre, special needs and also private practice. After much reflection on this journey, I have come to realize that the convergence of three seemingly different aspects of my own life – personal, spiritual and professional – into a symbiotic union is not accidental, but rather an evolutionary and natural progression for me. I have moved from awareness about self towards awareness about the relationship between self and others, and then from awareness about self and others towards transcending self and benefiting others.

Having been, myself, a witness to the immense benefit of art and Buddhism in my own life and seeing how together they helped me to heal and overcome many personal demons, I began to appreciate how they can work in complementary fashion and serve as an effective curative process which can lead an individual towards a journey of self-discovery and healing. Inspired by this realization and belief, over the last two years I have tried to develop these intervention models which seek complementary elements and strategies in art therapy practice. I am glad to say I have yielded very positive results both in individual and group settings. As an art therapist, I wish to explore newer possibilities as my understanding of the human mind and condition grows and changes over time. I will refine my practice by examining my intervention models and verifying their efficacy and theoretical basis.

References

Beer, R. (2004) *The Encyclopedia of Tibetan Symbols and Motifs.* Chicago, IL: Serindia Publications.

Dalai Lama (1995) *The World of Tibetan Buddhism: An Overview of Its Philosophy and Practice.* Sommerville: Wisdom.

Dalai Lama (2003) *A Collaboration Between Science and Religion.* Available at www.dalailama. com/messages/buddhism/science-and-religion, accessed on 4 November 2011.

Dzogchen Ponlop Rinpoche (1992) *A Science of Mind* [Online]. Available at www. ecobuddhism.org/index.php/download_file/-/view/161/l, accessed on 4 November 2011.

Fields, R. (2009) *Welcoming the Psychology Field to the 'Mindfulness Movement'.* Available at http://recoveryview.com/2009/04/welcoming-the-psychology-field-to-the-%E 2%80%9Cmindfulness-movement-%E2%80%9C/, accessed on 4 November 2011.

Fischer, Z.N. (2004) *Working with Emotions (Talk 2 of 7)*. Available at www.everydayzen. org/index.php?Itemid=27&option=com_teaching&topic=Emotions&sort=title& studyguide=true&task=viewTeaching&id=text-280-142, accessed 26 December 2010.

Jung, C.G. (1989) *Memories, Dreams, Reflections*, 4th edn. New York, NY: Vintage Book Edition.

Kabat-Zinn, J. (2005) *Full Catastrophe Living*. New York, NY: Bantam Dell.

McNiff, S. (1998) *Art-Based Research*. London: Jessica Kingsley Publishers.

Norbu, C.N. (1992) *Dream Yoga and the Practice of Natural Light*. New York, NY: Snow Lion.

Siegel, J.D. (2007) *Reflections on the Mindful Brain*. New York, NY: W.W. Norton.

The Mind and Life Institute (MLI) (n.d.) *History*. Available at www.mindandlife.org/ about/history/, accessed on 4 November 2011.

Watson, G. (2001) 'Buddhism meets Western science.' *Park Ridge Center Bulletin 19*. Available at www.parkridgecenter.org/Page483.html, accessed on 26 December 2010.

Chapter 11

Focusing-Oriented Art Therapy and Experiential Collage Work
History and Development in Japan

Laury Rappaport, Akira Ikemi and Maki Miyake

Focusing-Oriented Art Therapy (FOAT) and Experiential Collage Work (ECW) integrates Gendlin's (1981, 1996) Focusing approach with visual art. FOAT was created by Rappaport (1988, 1993, 1998, 2006, 2008, 2010), an art therapist in the United States, who synthesized Gendlin's Focusing with art therapy for a period of 30 years with a variety of clients in different treatment contexts. Ikemi (Ikemi, 2011; Ikemi *et al.*, 2007), a clinical psychologist, developed ECW out of his attempt to incorporate collage into Focusing. Rappaport and Ikemi are both Focusing Coordinators with The Focusing Institute in NY. The International Focusing Conference sponsored by The Focusing Institute became the vehicle for Rappaport and Ikemi to learn about each other's work. In addition to Rappaport and Ikemi, there have been Focusers integrating art into their practice (Ikemi *et al.*, 2007; Leijssen, 1992; Marder, 1997; Neagu, 1988; Tsuchie, 2003; Yuba and Murayama, 1988), and arts therapists using Focusing in their work (Knill, 2004; Knill, Levine and Levine, 2005; Merkur, 1997; Rappaport, 1988, 1993, 1998). This chapter describes the historical background of Focusing developed by Gendlin (1981, 1996) and its attunement to Japanese culture, along with an overview of FOAT and ECW with examples of their application to training and psychotherapy in Japan.

Focusing

Focusing is a psychotherapeutic and self-help approach developed by Gendlin (1981, 1996), a philosopher and psychologist, based on research that he conducted with Carl Rogers during the 1960s on what led to psychotherapy's effectiveness. After analyzing hundreds of therapy transcripts, they discovered that the success of the therapy did not correlate with the therapist's theoretical orientation, the content of what the client spoke about, or the therapist's technique. Instead, they found that the crucial factor was *how* the person spoke.

For example, clients might say that they had a "weird" dream. When psychotherapists ask how the dream was "weird," a client may say, "Oh, it was just some weird dream," and go no further. Other clients may listen more attentively within, noticing that the word "weird" is insufficient to carry the sense of the dream. The dream may have a sensed quality of scary, strange, and yet familiar, deep, and so forth, that cannot be expressed easily with a single word. These latter clients are tapping into a sense of the whole dream, which is bodily felt—such as a sense of something cramped in the chest while they talk about the dream. Often, these clients pause between words to check how their own words resonate with their bodily sensed experience.

Gendlin (1981) termed the phrase *felt sense* to explain this deeper bodily sense that some clients naturally accessed in their own speaking, describing it as "A bodily experience of a situation or person or event. An internal aura that encompasses everything you feel and know about a given subject at a given time" (pp.32–33). In order to teach people how to access the felt sense, Gendlin (1981) developed Focusing. Gendlin (1996) further developed Focusing-Oriented Psychotherapy (FOT) as a theoretical and practice application of Focusing to psychotherapy. In FOT, attention is paid to the quality of the relationship, the safety of the client, listening, and the interspersing of Focusing attuned to the experiential process of the client. According to Mary Hendricks-Gendlin, "Focusing was pretty much international from the start" (personal communication, 2011).

As of April 2011, Japan has 110 Certified Focusing Professionals/ Therapists, the largest number of Focusing professionals in any one country outside North America. How did Focusing get so firmly rooted in Japan, along with newer interests in FOAT and ECW? This question may be answered from two perspectives: the history of the academic climate in Japan in regard to psychotherapy, and the attunement of Focusing with Japanese culture.

History of academic climate in Japan in relation to psychotherapy

Client Centered Therapy (CCT) was already well known in Japan, and some Japanese professors who studied CCT (such as Professor Takao Murase) developed an interest in Gendlin's work. They started to translate Gendlin's articles on psychotherapy in the early 1960s (Gendlin, 1966), much before the book *Focusing* first came out in 1978. Since these professors had graduate students, many of whom eventually became the next generation of professors, research into Gendlin's psychotherapy, and subsequently Focusing, began and continued in academia. Currently more than 20 of the Certified Focusing Professionals in Japan work as full-time faculty in various universities across the country; more teach as adjunct faculty. Thus, through Japanese universities, the Rogers–Gendlin "lineage" continues to be taught and published.

Focusing and Japanese culture

Academic history, however, cannot account for the popularity of Focusing in Japan by itself. Why were the first generation professors inclined to study Gendlin's psychotherapy in the first place? Several areas of attunement between Japanese culture and Focusing can be elaborated.

Japanese culture is rich in artistic expression. From the art of tea to haiku poetry, bonsai, woodblock prints (ukioe), etc., Japanese culture values art, much more so than intellectual reasoning. One does not have to be Japanese to name some of the art forms developed in Japan, but when asked to name a prominent Japanese philosopher, an ordinary Japanese person will probably be unable to name a single one. It might even be said that reason or "rationale" comes second only, while the *sense* is primary in daily life in Japan. People who deduce their views and actions with reason are said to be "*rikutsu-poi*" (overly rational) and they do not appeal to others. Thus, the Focusing process of expressing the implicitly felt sense, whether in art form or in language, is familiar to most people in Japan. Both in Focusing and art expression, the expression process follows from sensed experience, not from formal logic.

The Japanese language has many expressions about the body that signify feelings. The body is often seen as the locale of deeper knowing. For example, the expression "*muné ni té wo atété kiité goran*" (put your hands on your chest and ask inside), which is often used today as a reprimand to those who rationalize their misbehavior, shows that the chest knows more than the rationalizations. "*Hara ga tatsu*" (to get angry) can be translated literally as "the gut forms (or stands out)", denoting that anger is a bodily felt experience. There is an expression for a type of a fool who is always in a hurry and cannot get things right. They are called "*ma nuké*," which literally means "space fallen off." Japanese people think that a person needs to be with the *ma*, in other words "clearing a space," a procedure in Focusing which, as shown below, comes naturally in Japanese culture. As can be seen, both Focusing and the arts resonate with Japanese culture. The following section describes the development of FOAT and ECW, with a basic overview and examples that demonstrate their affinity to aspects of Japanese culture previously described.

FOAT and ECW in Japan

When Rappaport learned Focusing in 1977, she was aware that artmaking naturally accessed what Gendlin termed the "felt sense." While creating art, the felt sense is engaged through the use of the body. For example, the hand, arm, and torso are engaged while painting, drawing, or sculpting. The felt sense implicitly informs color and material choices, guides the development of an image, unfolds answers, and knows when the art is complete. Focusing added something that Rappaport did not receive in her training as an art therapist. It added a mindfulness aspect—bringing a friendly, welcoming attitude toward the bodily felt sense and listening to it. Gendlin (1996) named this the "Focusing Attitude" and described its importance: "We might not like what we hear from the felt sense, but we want to be friendly to the messenger...and glad about its arrival" (p.55). Focusing provided a practice approach that helped Rappaport learn how to listen deeply to clients, to help clients access their inner knowing, and to navigate the moment-by-moment process of the client.

The root of bringing FOAT to Japan was the 2005 International Focusing Conference in Canada. At Rappaport's workshop, there were more Japanese Focusers than North Americans. Spontaneously, Mako Hikasa, Focusing Coordinator and Professor at Taisho University, translated. However, pairs were formed between Japanese and North American participants where artmaking provided a cross-cultural communication for connection and empathy. This embodied and aesthetic knowing resonated with many of the cultural aspects previously described. Miyake, a Focusing Trainer in the workshop, was studying at Kansai University with Ikemi. Out of their mutual interests in Focusing and visual art expression, a rich collaboration ensued resulting in the

Japanese translation of Rappaport's book and subsequent lectures and training on FOAT by Rappaport throughout Japan (Rappaport 2009a, 2009b).

ECW can be traced to the development of collage therapy in Japan. The works of the late Professor Hayao Kawai (Kyoto University), a Jungian therapist, was influential throughout Japanese clinical psychology. He introduced sand-play therapy to Japan as a way of working with children. Since sand-play required many materials, Professor Hiroyuki Moritani (1988) thought of using collage as an alternate form of sand-play, and reported the use of collage in psychotherapy. Subsequently, a "collage therapy" developed in Japan and gained popularity as collage tended to be a preferred medium of art for those who felt they were not competent with drawing. Ikemi, a Focusing Coordinator in Japan, started to experiment with collage, as several of his students introduced collage therapy to him. However, when he and his colleagues reviewed the literature on collage therapy, it came to his attention that the client's own sense of meaning of the collage was not given much attention in the literature. Collage tended to be used as a psychological assessment, and in therapy the therapist's interpretation of the collage was frequently reported. To reinstall the client's own experience of the collage, he and his colleagues formulated a Focusing-oriented approach to collage, ECW. ECW is known and practiced among Focusing professionals in Japan, in several universities and in the corporate mental health programs for managers. Despite a publication by Yano (2010), among mainstream clinical psychologists ECW is still confused with "collage therapy."

Focusing-Oriented Art Therapy (FOAT)

Foundational principles of FOAT include: therapeutic presence, listening, attending to safety, grounding, and the unique clinical needs of each client. In FOAT, one can either begin with Focusing or artmaking.

BASIC STEPS OF FOAT

When beginning with Focusing, the felt sense leads to artmaking. When beginning with artmaking, Focusing can assist with the art process and accessing meaning. A basic step is to begin with the Focusing Attitude (being friendly and welcoming) toward a felt sense of an experience, see if there is a "handle/symbol" as an image (or word, phrase, gesture, or sound), and express it in art. Note that "handle" or "symbol" is derived from Gendlin (1981).

This process of listening to the felt sense and seeing whether there is an image that matches it is the source and inspiration for art-making. FOAT trainings often begin with helping participants to have an experiential understanding of the Focusing Attitude. The following Focusing instructions help to bring mindful awareness toward the felt sense:

> Take a few deep breaths inside to your body…being friendly and accepting to whatever is happening within right now [Focusing Attitude]. Ask inside, how would I like to treat myself that would be kinder, gentler, more compassionate or accepting… (pause). Allow the body to let you know… Sense how it would feel for you to treat yourself this way… See if there is an image—or word, phrase, gesture, or sound [handle/symbol]—that matches the inner felt sense of how it would feel… When you're ready, choose art materials that express the felt sense of what it would feel like to treat yourself with the attitude that came to you.

In response, one participant shared the following (Figure 11.1):

> I always hold myself to a high standard and often feel like I'm not good enough. During the Focusing, the word acceptance came. I had a sense inside of melting…and resting in softness. My heart felt light. Using the art materials, I surrounded my heart with feathers and soft materials. I placed stars around with one a star in the center of my heart—letting me know that I am okay just as I am…acceptance.

When clients are inclined to begin with art, Focusing can be integrated afterwards. For example, after clients create art, they can be guided to bring a friendly attitude toward the art and inner experience, access a felt sense of the art, and then see if there is a word, phrase, image, gesture, or sound (handle/symbol) that matches it. This is a useful way to bring mindful awareness to the process, ground the experience in the body, add a title to art, and unfold meaning.

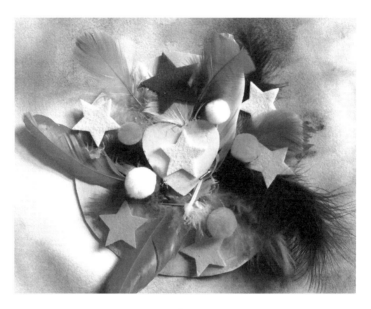

Figure 11.1 *Melting and resting in softness*

FOAT APPROACHES

Rappaport (2009a) adapted Gendlin's Focusing to create three basic approaches.

CLEARING A SPACE WITH ART

The client identifies the issues that are in the way of feeling "all fine" and imagines placing them at a distance outside of the body. Imagery is incorporated in helping to set the issues at a distance that feels right in order to "clear the space." For example, the client might imagine wrapping each issue up in a package and placing it at a comfortable distance, or putting a concern or problem on a boat and letting it float out on a lake. Art is incorporated in order to concretize and symbolize the felt sense of the issues being set aside. After clearing the issues, the client gets a felt sense of the "all fine place" and symbolizes it in art. The following is an example from the Clearing a Space with Art Workshop in Japan:

> Take a few deep breaths inside to your body…being friendly and accepting to whatever is happening within right now. Check inside and ask, "What's between me and feeling 'all fine' right now?" As each concern comes up, just notice it,

without going into it. Imagine wrapping each concern up and setting it at a distance from you. As you put each thing aside, sense how it feels inside. Check again…"Except for all of that, I'm all fine." Once you set aside the concerns or stressors, notice how you are inside. See if there is an image that matches your inner felt sense of the "all fine place."

A participant used twisted papers to represent her concerns. She shared:

> I felt so many concerns that I could not manage. I put them aside using the twisted papers. After, I found that there was a hidden space at the center of the art (Figure 11.2). I felt a space, like a Tatami room, where I could lay down. While I was making the art, the Tatami room suddenly felt like "my hideout." I covered the room with a sheet of paper to keep it hidden and protected (Figure 11.3). Although I am in a difficult situation in my life, I can now allow myself to go to this Tatami room. I feel a sense of ease when I imagine that I am in the room (tears). From here, I can see what's going on outside but no one would know I am here! How exciting!

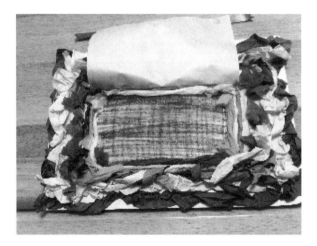

Figure 11.2 *Tatami room with hidden space*

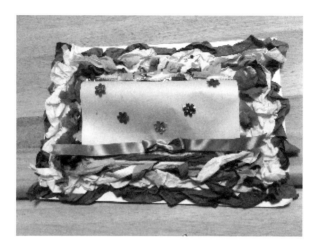

Figure 11.3 *"All fine place." Tatami room protected space*

Clearing a space with art helps clients to have an experiential knowing that there is a place of inherent wholeness within. At first, the participant was overwhelmed with her concerns. As the participant set her issues aside during clearing a space, she found a protected, safe space (Tatami room) where then she could find an inner sense of ease. A change, or "felt shift" (Gendlin, 1981), can be seen as her state changed from overwhelmed with difficulty to excited. Clearing a space with art is useful for stress reduction, as well as an entry point to the other two approaches.

THEME-DIRECTED *FOAT*

A theme-directed approach is primarily used with groups, in which topics related to the groups needs, such as strengths, fears, hopes, life balance, and so forth, are explored. It can also be used with individuals and couples to address specific themes. The following is an example exercise:

> Take a few deep breaths into your body... Become aware of something in your life that has been a source of strength [e.g. person, something from nature, spiritual, etc.]. As you bring it into your awareness, notice how it feels in your body. See if there's an image that matches or acts like a handle for the felt sense. Check it for a sense of rightness. When you have it, use the art materials to create your felt sense image.

When offering the theme of a "source of strength," one participant shared:

> My source of strength is my grandmother (Figure 11.4). She was always there for me and gave me great love. Whenever I go through a dark or difficult time, I imagine her with me. When I focused, I sensed her quiet strength and love within me. I felt grounded and solid in my body...in the midst of a difficulty that I have now.

Many participants remarked that it felt good to focus on a positive theme that can be useful for working on issues.

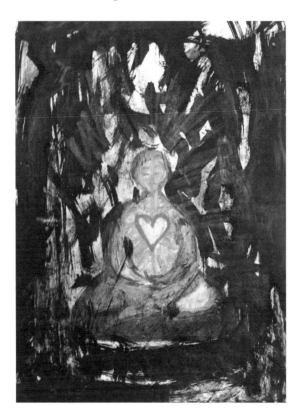

Figure 11.4 *Source of strength*

FOCUSING-ORIENTED ART PSYCHOTHERAPY

In focusing-oriented art psychotherapy, art therapy and parts of Gendlin's Focusing method are interspersed during a psychotherapy encounter.

The session may begin with Focusing on a specific issue or beginning with art and then integrating the Focusing process. There is generally an alternation among Focusing, artmaking, sharing, listening, Focusing, etc. Focusing-oriented art psychotherapy is primarily applied to individual and couples' therapy where the issues arise out of the client's experiencing and the orientation is toward understanding and living differently. Although Ikemi's ECW is its own method, it also serves as an example of Rappaport's focusing-oriented art psychotherapy.

Experiential collage work

There are two parts to ECW—creating a collage followed by Focusing and listening. In the collage-making process, clients choose a sheet of colored construction that matches how they feel at the moment. Next, they browse through magazines and make clippings of pictures and/ or words that appeal to them. After sorting through the images and/or words, clients place them on the paper, sensing the right arrangement, and then glue them onto the construction paper to complete the collage. In the second part, Focusing and listening are integrated into the process in order to help clients explore the meaning of their collage.

As an example, the client chose a light blue colored sheet of paper and placed the following: tea plantation, trees with children, two sake cups and a bottle of sake, a poem in calligraphy, pot of food, mountains and sky, hot spring, indoor bath, and mountain from above (Figure 11.5). The Japanese words in the center are translated in English as "Holiday for adults" (horizontal) and "Finding the forgotten self" (vertical). The vertical words on the lower right corner translate as "Wanting time to spend for myself." The caption on the trunk of the center tree reads "Encounter yourself."

In Part 2, the client shared reflections about the collage while the therapist responded with experiential listening and Focusing suggestions in order to help the client access a personal meaning. The following transcript highlights how experiential listening and Focusing are interspersed within the client's sharing about his collage:

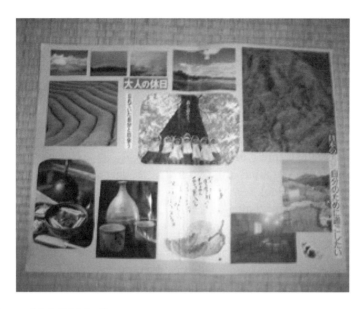

Figure 11.5 *ECW collage*

CL1: I haven't taken a vacation with my family for a couple of years. I mean, I do feel the need to take a break, I really do. But, I just don't feel like traveling with my family.

TH1: There's something within you that makes you feel like...not wanting to travel with your family [listening].

CL2: Yes, but I do want to go alone. Maybe it's too much pressure from work, but I don't feel like traveling with my family...and it makes me feel like, maybe I don't really love them.

TH2: There is a lot of pressure from work, and then there is this not wanting to travel with your family. You even begin to wonder if you love them enough? [listening].

CL3: Well...yes, I do feel the pressure and wanting to be alone.

TH3: Let's see now, I wonder how all of this feels in your body? As you sense the whole collage, see how you feel in the middle of the body, in the throat, chest, abdomen area... [guiding to access a felt sense].

CL4: Uhm...there's some sadness there. It's like a shrinking feeling in my chest [felt sense—is in the body].

TH4: There's a shrinking feeling there in the chest, and it's sadness? [listening—reflecting the felt sense]. Is sadness or shrinking the right word for it? [resonating for the expression (symbol/handle) with the felt sense].

CL5: Yes, yes… It's sadness there [symbol/handle].

TH5: See if you can be friendly to the sadness [Focusing Attitude]. Stay with the sadness for a moment and see what comes from there [listening to the felt sense].

CL6: Oh! You know what? Look at this picture…here of the two sake cups. I'm wanting to be alone and yet there are two cups. And what comes to my mind just now is that I want to have sake with my father. And look here! There's a poem here and the last line begins with the word "father."

More came from the felt sense of sadness. The client said that his father had died of a traffic accident three years earlier. It was quite a shock, because his father had been totally healthy until that morning when his life was suddenly taken. His mother fell ill immediately afterwards and died a few months later. The client now recalled that he had no time to mourn the loss of his father, since his mother's condition and subsequent death overshadowed the mourning process for his father. After telling this story of his father's death, the client realized that the picture of the tea plantation in the middle left looked identical to a place where he and his father used to drive when he was in college. Their car had a flat tire and couldn't move out of a tea plantation, which looked exactly like the one in the picture. He didn't notice this connection during the making of the collage. The client now realized that he needed time to mourn the loss of his father before he could move on to vacationing with his family.

As seen in the ECW, initially clients usually do not know why they may be choosing certain images; however, there is an implicit knowing in choosing images that have a personal meaning. Instead of the therapist "interpreting" meaning from the collage, clients explore their own sense of meaning as they speak about the collage. The therapist interweaves experiential listening and Focusing in relation to the client's unfolding experiential process in order to help the client access the meaning within themselves. As demonstrated in the example, the therapist listened to the client about the images and invited the client to notice the felt sense that accompanied the collage. As the client accessed the sadness, the felt meaning became explicit. From the "sadness" came the client's understanding that he needed time to mourn the loss of his father, which implied a new way of living his vacation.

Conclusion

As can be seen, Focusing, FOAT, and ECW are naturally attuned to the Japanese culture. FOAT has had an impact on Focusing professionals, because many of them had been experimenting with expressing the bodily felt sense through art, rather than through words. However, since most of the Focusing professionals are psychologists and not art therapists, they do not have a sufficient background in art therapy to establish their experimentations as a specific method of practice. For example, the Japanese Association of Psychopathology of Expression and Arts Therapy with approximately a 1000 members has a mixed membership consisting mostly of medical professionals. Japan's receptiveness to FOAT is therefore twofold: as a new form of Focusing for Focusing professionals/therapists and as providing a knowledge base in art therapy.

We look forward to the rich exchange of FOAT and ECW with other clinical art therapy and psychotherapy programs, associations, and individuals.

References

Gendlin, E. (1966) *Taiken Katei to Shinriryouhou* [Experiencing and Psychotherapy—A Collection of Papers] (Trans. Takao Murase) Tokyo: Natsumesha.

Gendlin, E.T. (1981) *Focusing*. New York, NY: Bantam Books. [Originally published in 1978 from New York, Everest House.]

Gendlin, E.T. (1996) *Focusing-Oriented Psychotherapy: A Manual of the Experiential Method*. New York, NY: Guilford Press.

Ikemi, A. (2011) 'Empowering the implicitly functioning relationship.' *Person-Centered and Experiential Psychotherapies 10*, 1, 28–42.

Ikemi, A., Yano, K., Miyake, M. and Matsuoka, S. (2007) 'Experiential collage work: Exploring meaning in collage from a focusing-oriented perspective.' *Journal of Japanese Clinical Psychology 25*, 4, 464–475.

Knill, P. (2004) *Minstrels of Soul: Intermodal Expressive Therapy*. Toronto: Palmerston Press.

Knill, P., Levine, S. and Levine, E. (2005) *Principles and Practice of Expressive Therapy: Towards a Therapeutic Aesthetics*. London: Jessica Kingsley Publishers.

Leijssen, M. (1992) 'Experiential focusing through drawing.' *The Folio 11*, 3, 35–40.

Marder, D. (1997) 'Sarah: Focusing and play therapy with a six-year-old child.' *The Folio 16*, 1–2, 75–80.

Merkur, B. (1997) 'Focusing using art with adolescents.' *The Folio 16*, 1–2, 51–54.

Moritani, H. (1988) 'Shinri-ryouhou ni Okeru Collage no Riyou' [On the Use of Collage in Psychotherapy]. *Psychiatria et Neurologica Japonica 90*, 5, 450.

Neagu, G. (1988) 'The focusing technique with children and adolescents.' *The Folio 7*, 4, 1–26.

Rappaport, L. (1988) 'Focusing and art therapy.' *The Focusing Connection 5*, 3, 1–2.

Rappaport, L. (1993) 'Focusing with art and creative movement: A method for stress management.' *The Focusing Connection 10*, 2, 1–3.

Rappaport, L. (1998) 'Focusing and art therapy: Tools for working through post-traumatic stress disorder.' *The Folio 17*, 1, 36–40.

Rappaport, L. (2006) 'Clearing a space: Expressing the wholeness within using art' (unpublished article). Available at www.focusing.org/arts_therapy.html#art_therapy, accessed on 21 November 2011.

Rappaport, L. (2008) 'Focusing-oriented art therapy.' *The Folio 21*, 1, 139–155.

Rappaport, L. (2009a) *Focusing-Oriented Art Therapy: Accessing the Body's Wisdom and Creative Intelligence.* London: Jessica Kingsley Publishers.

Rappaport, L. (2009b) *Focusing-Oriented Art Therapy* (Trans. A. Ikemi and M. Miyake) Tokyo: Seishin Shobo [in Japanese].

Rappaport, L. (2010) 'Focusing-oriented art therapy and trauma.' *Journal of Person-Centered and Experiential Psychotherapies 9*, 2, 128–143.

Tsuchie, S. (2003) 'Our internal weather: Staying in focus.' *The Focusing Institute Newsletter 3*, 1, 1.

Yano, K. (2010) 'Experiential collage work and the creation of meaning.' *Japanese Journal of Humanistic Psychology 28*, 1, 63–75 [in Japanese].

Yuba, N. and Murayama, S. (1988) 'Clearing a space with drawing in play therapy.' *The Folio 7*, 1, 11–22.

PART 4

Role of Art Traditions

Chapter 12

Landscape of the Mind

Evelyna Liang Kan

In the beginning:
There is 'Qi', and it is called the GREAT.
There is 'Dao', and it is the WAY.

Ever since I was old enough to hold a brush, I started to scribble with ink-wash on paper. I enjoyed being able to make marks and leave my sign. I learned to draw character words when I was two and a half and later I found out that I was actually creating my own type of Chinese calligraphy. I started to paint in the Chinese way when I was studying in Canada. Holding a brush in my hand and drawing with ink seemed so natural that it never occurred to me that it might not be. The brush, the ink and the rice paper are the tools that are dearest to my heart, and with them I started to paint my imaginary landscape of home. I enjoyed landscape painting, for it provided me with a sense of escape, an escape into the imaginary land where there is peace. Not being able to return to China in my university days made me yearn for all things Chinese. I started to search for the meaning of being Chinese and thus began my quest.

Brief history of Chinese painting

In his historical review, Lee (1964) points out that when one encounters Chinese painting or Chinese art we are reminded of the importance of being able to work and achieve *qi* of heaven and earth. Qi is the aim of most Chinese artists, and the concept also applies to the character and virtue of the artist. As far back as the Jin Dynasty, the famous painter Gu Kaizhi (顧愷之) (c. 344–406 ad) was highly praised as one of the best artists of his era, and it was commented that the figures he created were as vivid as real people, as if they could actually jump out of the painting and become alive.

From the 6th century to the 8th century, when the themes of painting shifted from figurative to landscape and calligraphic strokes, the union between the painted visual form and the spirit and virtue of the artist became emphasized. To paint nature is also to paint and re-create the spirit of nature qi, that the artist should hold, and convey through his brush. To the Chinese mind, nature itself is symbolic. All creation typifies something higher, and the clearer the design the more apparent the purpose.

As early as the 6th century, art historian and critic Xie He (Hsieh Ho 謝赫) stated that the first principle in Chinese painting is '*Qi Yun Sheng Dong*' (氣韻生動). This phrase is translated as 'breath energy and rhythmic vitality' or 'breath, resonance and vital force'. The other five principles are disciplined brushwork, proper representation of objects, specific coloration, good composition and copying of old masters.

Meaning of qi: Breath energy

Qi, as the most important of all principles, literally means 'air' or 'breath'. In old Chinese pictographic form (Table 12.1), the character qi originally had the shape of a rising cloud, comprising three horizontal strokes, in which the bottom stroke represents the earth, the middle one mist, and the top stroke cloud. It almost looks like the character 'three' (三) and can quite easily be confused with it. Over time, it developed so the top stroke curved slightly upward to the left and the bottom stroke curved slightly downward to the right. The character had the meaning of 'cloud qi' – the rising vapours that gather to form the cloud. Qi is air, something that cannot always be seen, but through its changes can be sensed, experienced and understood (Zhang and Rose, 2001). As the written character and meaning of qi evolved over time, it took on the meaning of breathing (xi 吸). Later, the character 'rice' (米) was added at the bottom inside part to form the present character, qi (氣). To eat (吃 chi), actually has the same phonetic sound as qi.

Table 12.1 *Evolution of qi character*

三	⩴	气
'earth, mist, cloud'	'cloud qi'	'breathing in and out'

This evolution shows qi is not only vapour, but is also an essential nutritional substance. We eat rice to give nourishment to the body. We need air to maintain life. We breathe in and breathe out in a continuous and ongoing flow. We need oxygen (air) in our blood stream to circulate around the body, to return to the original intake place for exchange with new input. All kinds of living creatures, including flora, need air to survive. In the physical world, both air and food are vital sources of energy. Therefore, qi is the matter that gives us life. It is the 'life force' and 'energy source' and is that which flows through all things (Figures 12.1a and 12.1b). It can be found in any material substance and is the spirit embedded in all creation. Qi is also like the wind; we might not be able to see it but it is upon us and we know it exists by the way it affects our physical surroundings. Chuang Tsu (1974) wrote:

> The Universe has a cosmic breath. Its name is wind. Sometimes it is not active; but when it is, angry howls rise from ten thousand openings. Have you ever heard a roaring gale? (p.20)

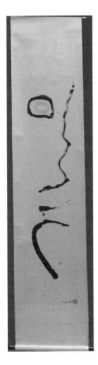

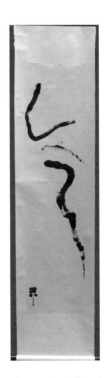

Figure 12.1a *One breath*   **Figure 12.1b** *Qi*

Qi is like water in that it can flow to wherever it is needed and is always in a continuous changing phase of its own cycles; it can fill any vessel in which it is contained and takes on its shape. Pour it into another container and it will change its shape and form. The new shape and form is thus the exact copy of the object. Water, in all its different variations and phases, is consequently one of the most important themes in Chinese landscape painting (Willis, 1987). According to the great Chinese philosopher Laozi (Lao Tzu 老子), qi is *Dao* (道) or the 'Way'. He (1972) wrote:

> Something mysteriously formed,
> Born before heaven and earth.
> In the silence and the void,
> Standing alone and unchanging,
> Ever present and in motion.
> Perhaps it is the mother of ten thousand things.
> I do not know its name.
> Call it Tao.
> For lack of a better word, I call it great.
> (Tao Te Ching, Chapter 25, lines 1–9)

Qi is the direct spirit of Dao as it dwells in form and moves through reality. Dao, in its original written form, represents a person's face (首), with hair flying, as when one is in motion and running (走) along a path (道). Thus the meaning of Dao is simply to 'follow the path', or to put it another way:

> To follow Tao is to follow
> The breath (qi) of the world. (Deng, 1996, p.14)

It also has the meaning of the divine intelligence, the principle, doctrine, the word and to speak the truth. It is very similar to the Christian doctrine; as Jesus said, 'I am the way and the truth and the life' (Holy Bible, John 14:6). Qi is believed to be the spirit and essence of every being, and Dao is before being: the origin and basis of all creation.

Chinese artists believe that a painting is not only a graphic sign that conveys meaning – the meaning of life – but is more. Although a work of art is a physical mark of the artist, through the practice of art, be it in painting, calligraphy, music, dance or poetry, one can be connected with the qi of heaven and earth and attain harmony in life as well. Qi should dwell in the creator of Art. Qi is the mother of all things. Qi gives birth and nourishment. All humans are born from qi and continuously receive qi from nature. All beings in nature are protectors, carriers and companions of qi. They bear witness to qi as well. Qi is revealed in man's virtue as the link between heaven and earth and humanity.

Meaning of Yun (韻): Rhythmic resonance

The second word in the phrase 'Qi Yun Sheng Dong' is *Yun*. It is defined as 'rhythmic resonance', the lingering resonance when all else has ceased. It is like the moment of silence or the pause in music when the notes have stopped, but the music continues to ring in your ears and in your mind. It also describes the essence or the good memories that one leaves behind and the memorable good virtue of benevolent men.

When the two words qi and yun are combined, another dimension of meaning appears. Huang Yueh (黄鉞), painter, writer and seal artist of the late 18th century, made reference to the meaning of qi yun in his 'Twenty-four Qualities of Chinese Painting'. He wrote:

> Of the Six Principles, Spirit Resonance is of first importance.
> Idea leads Brush. Wonder beyond the painting!
> Like melody lingering on strings; like fog fading into mist.
> Heaven's fresh wind, vibrating waves...
> The apparent, large or small, becomes intangible, fluid.
> Read ten thousand books,
> Something may be revealed. (Tseng, 1963, p.8)

To attain qi yun in one's work, the traditional Chinese artists believed that it was important to look within oneself. The spirit of art is buried in one's subconscious. For the artist to find it, one must search for it and excavate it by diligent effort. It is akin to arousing one's creative potential through soul searching.

It is also important for one to master the tool – the brush – to use it to reach the level of qi yun. Good brushwork comes from calligraphy. They are two inseparable elements from the same source. Both require skill and disciplined handling. To control the brush (*pi* 筆), be disciplined and learn from the old masters, yet be able to stir and turn the wrist and arm and fly free to create one's own method. One must hold the ink (*mo* 墨) in the brush and make a dry land (line) or vaporous mist in one single sweep. The line and rhythm of the brushwork are considered to be the vehicle carrying the qi. The energy from within the artist is transmitted through the body onto the brush tip, then to the rice paper. Consequently, in order to make a wonderful painting with the brush, first one should handle it as in calligraphy. Second, one must learn from nature, observe nature's own rhythmic movement (as all ancient masters did), and take notes from the masters' ways and methods. Third, when you have grasped the first two principles, empty your mind of these rules and be prepared to improvise. Do not be bound by limitation of any kind; be your own master and free. Then qi yun will come naturally.

In my own experience, I loved to hold the brush and create marks that might not mean anything at all. Only later did I find that I was actually moving the brush with my mind's eye, the spirit and energy from nature. I drew lines up and down the paper, swirled them around in the ever rippling pattern of water, splashed the ink and watched it bleed into familiar patterns. I used the brush to create patches of ink and colour to record my thoughts of happiness and joy. It is the artwork that plays within and between the conscious and the unconscious mind. It is intangible, the idea or concept that is of most importance, yet it also requires knowledge and skill. Even though critics in the past often thought that to be able to attain qi yun in one's work was akin to receiving a gift from heaven, it can be acquired by study or it may at least be developed through respect for nature and humanity. To be a great artist meant, after all, not only to have the gift, but also to possess the brush of a scholar.

Chinese landscape painting

Traditional Chinese artists believe that a landscape painting is like a mirror that reflects not only the natural scenery of mountain and water, but also the vibration of life, culminating in the movement of heaven and earth. The principle of 'Qi Yun Sheng Dong' posits that the artwork and its creator should bond together in the right spirit/energy of qi. *Sheng Dong* (生動), the last two words, mean 'vital force' or 'movement'. This vital energy of the artist process in creating an artwork should later be transferred to whomever is viewing the artwork. For example, a landscape painting that can move viewers and arouse in them an urge to dwell in such a landscape would be considered a successful artwork displaying qi yun sheng dong, for it can move the soul (Figure 12.2).

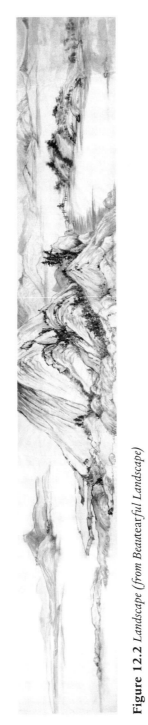

Figure 12.2 *Landscape (from Beautearful Landscape)*

This phenomenon can be applied to listening to a musical performance or watching a dance piece. The swift and slow movement, the dense and scattered spacing between each stroke and the repetitive lines all suggest a living body dancing in the wind. It is similar to composing music, as different notes and chords are required: accelerando and ritardando in the spacing of landscape elements, crescendos as in the piling up of the mountain ranges and diminuendos in the fading away into mist. Void or empty space is sometimes used to accentuate the moving forces, enabling the viewer to take a pause before or after a grand opening or finale.

When we say that the Chinese artist is creating a landscape painting, it is really not the true landscape that he is creating. He is creating his own images and idea of nature. He uses the landscape to pass on his belief; he creates a landscape for his mind and soul to take a rest. He is creating a personal space for escape in a world that is off balance. He will take the viewer with him using the landscape as the vehicle to transport to the inner realm of qi. The artist who created the work is guiding the viewer to his imaginary world, but at the pace of the viewer, as if in an interactive journey. The viewer can roll the painting scroll back and forth, pick his own scene, wander about, and trace the ins and outs and ups and downs of the mountainscape. He can stop any time he wishes only to continue the tour in perhaps a couple of hours, days, months or even years. The journey is both physical and virtual. It is a journey in time and space. The real journey involves looking up and down, left and right, rolling and unrolling or, if the painting is spread out in a gallery, walking back and forth. The journey is also in the mind. The viewer will be walking with the spirit of the artists, of the landscape he created, and of nature.

Contemporary use of qi and landscape

For the past years working both as a visual artist and a community arts practitioner, I use the form of traditional Chinese art for self-assurance and self-fulfilment. With this knowledge as my background, first I create paintings that serve to balance my own busy life, to let me escape into the imaginary world of the brushwork and be in touch with nature. Second, I share with the community I serve on how to use art to reach the mindful spirit of qi and understand the path and pattern of our own energy around and within us. Third, I offer art as a way for self-healing and a channel for my outcry for a battered society.

Big Water Comes...

In the year 2006, on Boxing Day (26 December), sad news of the South Asian tsunami shook the world. With the non-stop bombardment from the media, one became even more traumatized when viewing the repeated images. In an attempt to help myself, I started to paint my sorrow in a long scroll as if I was walking the sorrowful paths with those who lost members of their family. Pouring water and ink splashes onto the paper, I created chaos with red dye. I marked the pain, I heard the lament of a child and I recorded it in words.

A long scroll, *Big Water Comes...* (Figure 12.3), emerged where pain, loss and deliverance were evident. My hurt was being exposed to the outside and left to live in the open on the painted scroll. Every time I either heard more sad or comforting news of the tsunami, I unrolled the scroll and journeyed along the path to find peace again. Sometimes I added more to the work while sometimes I left a silent empty space, waiting for the next moment that will guide me to a fuller understanding of the event.

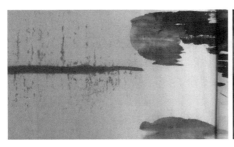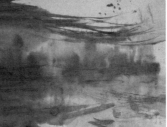

Figure 12.3 *Big Water Comes...*

Beautearful Landscape

I have been angered by news of contemporary man destroying the earth, replacing trees with artificial plastic ones along the riverbanks in scenic China, and constructing more and more unnecessary buildings while scourging and excavating ores and stones from beautiful hillsides. Pouring toxic waste and contaminating the land, I think the earth is weeping, in pain. I created a 120 foot long landscape painting in response to this world. In the past, Chinese artists might have used landscape painting as a way to attain peace, but in this painting I used it as a way to convey a message. It is a journey through an artist's eye, but in response to what we have done to nature.

I chose to copy Huang Gong Wang's (黃公望, 1269–1354) long hand scroll *Dwelling in the Fu-ch'un Mountain* (富春山居圖卷) of 1350 ad. I tried to erase my melancholy towards the modern age through copying. Every day, the act of painting consoled my sadness and alleviated my worries. The scroll became longer and longer to about 90 feet in length. I coloured the mountains and rivers with light colours – green, cyan, yellow. I dreamt of a peaceful and beautiful landscape. The reality is that times change, and landscapes change, too.

High-rise buildings stand tall beside the river, paddy terraces become golf clubs, man-made dams and artificial lakes begin to appear in our natural landscape. Mountains have been exploded to build houses and highways. Finally, my own *Beautiful Landscape*, transformed with cement, industrial dyes, bleaches, synthetic rubber, detergent, plastic tress and plastic cartoon figures, it became a landscape dedicated to modern people. After a series of rubbing, bleaching and colouring, the beautiful landscape collapsed and was torn into pieces. The bleach turned the scroll pale and irritated the senses. Tears were shed, hence *Beautearful Landscape*.

For the next couple of months I tried to mend all the torn pieces and patch all the cracks. At the very end of the scroll, I added another 30 feet of imaginary landscape of a world that I so wished for. The famous 16th-century monk artist Shi Tao (as cited in Ba Da and Shi Tao, 2004) once said:

> Landscape (nature) has given me the power to speak for them.
> Landscape arises from me, I arise from landscape, when our spirits meet, painting is the mark! (p.314)

I chose to use my art to be a spokesperson for our landscape. I asked the question, 'Can we save our earth?'

Time became my witness. I recorded the whole process and exhibited the work through a video installation alongside the tormented long scroll. I used this piece of artwork to arouse awareness. When visitors were watching the projection of the video on the ground, the moving images under their feet provided an unstable sensation (Figures 12.4a and 12.4b). Viewers felt the earth was shaking and weeping. My artwork guided their eyes and feet as they walked the path of what we have done to our earth. For those who had witnessed the digitized landscape torn right under their feet, I passed on my sorrow and anger. In the open area where I exhibited the long scroll, I encouraged everyone to walk slowly and bend down to view the work. I invited them to help replace the plastic plants with real shrubs. Children who came to my workshop during the exhibition even suggested putting soil on the painting and planting real grass.

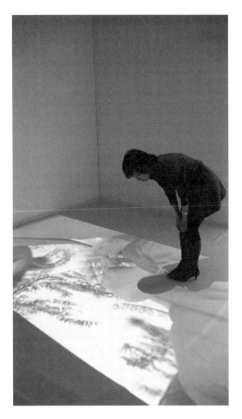

Figure 12.4a *Looking at the installation of Beautearful Landscape*

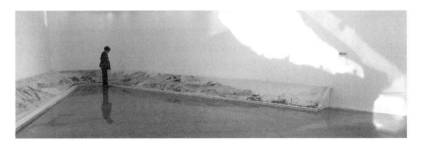

Figure 12.4b *Viewing the video projection of Beautearful Landscape*

I showed my landscape painting as it took place within a different perspective of time, and all the changes it made, from the past to the present and visions for the future. I left the viewers with their own interpretations and their own individual answers to my question. It is important that, in a painting, a viewer should allow for interpretation through imagination. A painting should never be fully painted and spatially defined. Whether it describes vast or empty space, it should be there for the viewer to meditate. It can be that of the invisible air or the void, just as much as the material substance; hence the spirit of qi works for both the viewer and the artist.

'thinking of Shui' (墨想水白)

Confucius (as cited in Chuang Tsu, 1974) said:

> Your will must be one. Do not listen with your ears but with your mind. Do not listen with your mind but with your vital energy. Ears can only hear, mind can only think, but vital energy is empty, receptive to all things. Tao abides in emptiness. Emptiness is the fasting of mind. (p.68)

Thus, empty spaces in a Chinese landscape painting are not empty but, on the contrary, represent the spirit of heaven and earth. To attain Dao, one has to be empty in order to receive fullness. For busy contemporary people, we rarely have time to look at the pattern and changes of time, let alone to find time to empty oneself for the quiet moment to listen to qi. In response, I created another piece of artwork to help people focus on the spirit of heaven and earth to seek Dao.

Again I used the long scroll format. At the beginning of the scroll, I copied the first two chapters of Ecclesiastes (the Holy Bible), from 'Emptiness is empty...all is empty' (1:1) to 'What do people gain from all the toil at which they toil under the sun...' (2:22). I copied the same two chapters six times and each time I started from the same spot. I dipped the brush in ink at each beginning sequence. When it dried up I only dipped the brush in water to moisten it and continued writing the verses. I continued this way until no more ink marks were visible. Next, I repeated a similar process by ink wash, six times again. I created a 70 foot long scroll; one end is darkened by writing and gradually fades into the nothingness of the original colour of the paper on the other end. One end is filled with continuous labour and calligraphic ink marks, while the other end is almost pure and untouched.

I installed the work in a dimly lit room and hung it from the ceiling, so that the ends faced each other on opposite walls to form a U-shape. The painting was randomly folded in the middle to create the feeling of the undulating mountain ranges from nature. I put two black lacquered bowls of water sitting on each side of the scroll where it started to curve up to the ceiling, one close to the darkened end and one to the untouched end. I turned on the faint sound of running water to create a quiet ambient atmosphere. With spotlights shone and focused onto the bowls of water, I invited viewers to write on the water. They were requested to kneel down in front of the bowl of water facing whichever end of the scroll they wanted and to write their own calligraphy on water (Figures 12.5a and 12.5b).

Many times visitors to the exhibition quietly concentrated on the movement of their brush and watched how the water moved. They did not seem to understand the connection of their actions with the scroll they were facing. When one started to aimlessly look around, it dawned on them. The writing they made in the water bowl formed reflective beautiful flickering lights on the untouched end of the scroll, whereas the darkened side absorbed the lights and remained black. In the empty spaces of the untouched scroll, one's energy and movement echoed back as dancing light. Each movement or stroke that one made was unique, as if in a direct intimate dialogue with nature. The spirit of qi is in evidence only when we empty all thoughts; then we can receive and see.

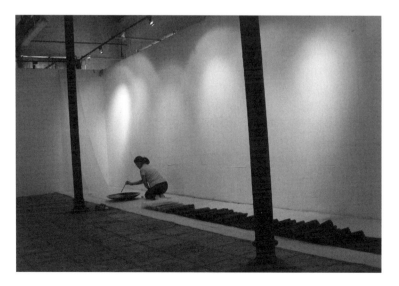

Figure 12.5a *'I write on white. Think of Shui'*

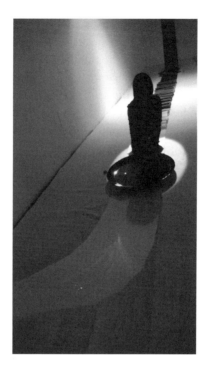

Figure 12.5b *Looking for light*

I titled this work:
   '*th*ink*ing of Shui*' (墨想水白)

> Meditation on Ink,
> Dialogue with water,
> Spirited inflection,
> Joyous resonance,
> Light,
> The most sublime!
> If
> There is no water; will Ink's five colours still exist?
> If there is no Ink, where will the voided space of water be?
> If
> There is no Light
> Then all is still in Chaos

Conclusion

Incorporating traditional Chinese art forms for contemporary concerns allowed me to reconcile my identity as a repatriated Chinese artist. In using nature imagery and elements of nature in my art, I call to mind how nature, for the Chinese, can be quite different from the Western view of wilderness, whereby the untouched virgin land should be controlled and subdued. Chinese philosophies regarded nature as the teacher from which humanity can learn. To learn from nature is to live in accord with the natural order of life, to follow the pattern and order of the universe. To attain qi in one's work, an artist has to prepare a tranquil heart, empty of desire and lust. In stillness the heart of the artist can become one with the elements of nature, the great creative forces of Dao – the true meaning of wholeness.

References

Ba Da and Shi Tao (2004) 'Rules by the Masters: Paintings and Calligraphies by Ba Da and Shi Tao, Collections of the Palace Museum and Shanghai Museum.' *Aomen yi shu bo wu guan.* Macau: Macau Museum of Art.

Chuang Tsu (1974) *Chuang Tsu: Inner Chapters* (Trans., G.-F. Feng and J. English) New York, NY: Vintage Books.

Deng, M.-D. (1996) *Everyday Tao: Living with Balance and Harmony.* New York, NY: HarperCollins.

The Holy Bible: New International Version (1984) Grand Rapids, MI: Zondervan.

Lao Tzu (1972) *Tao Te Ching* (Trans., G.-F. Feng and J. English) New York, NY: Vintage Books.

Lee, S.E. (1964) *A History of Far Eastern Art.* New York, NY: Harry N. Abrams.

Tseng, Y.-H. (1963) *Some Contemporary Elements in Classical Chinese Art.* Honolulu, HI: University of Hawaii Press.

Willis, B. (1987) *The Tao of Art: The Inner Meaning of Chinese Art and Philosophy.* London: Ebury Press.

Zhang, Y.H. and Rose, K. (2001) *A Brief History of Qi.* Brookline, MA: Paradigm.

Chapter 13

The Arts
A Unique Mantra for Healing

Shanta Serbjeet Singh

If there is a single window into the mysterious world of Indian art and aesthetics it is the traditional Indian holistic and cosmocentric vision of the world. It explains the relationship of the parts to the whole, of the multiple to the one, and of the finite to the infinite. Man acquires special significance not because he is the best and conquers nature, but because he is one amongst the many with a capacity for consciousness and ability to transcend pure physicality through psychic discipline.

This chapter (which is based on an address I gave in 2001 to the Fourth Asia Pacific Performing Arts Network Conference) seeks to connect the arts both with ancient Indian philosophical concepts and with health practices and concepts, as documented from the time of the Rig Veda. The four *Vedas*, variously placed at 3000 years before Christ, deal with the nature of phenomena, of the existence of man and other aspects of the vast cosmos. The oldest book that talks about the Indian performance arts, Sage Bharata's *Natya Shastra*, called the fifth *Veda*, after the four *Vedas* (between 200 bc and 200 ad), contains a vast treasury of written material which details the effect of the arts on the minutest and most microcosmic layers of the body.

At the end of my exploration of concepts drawn from both the Vedas and Ayurveda, the Indian science of health, as well as of later Sanskrit texts that elucidate the philosophy *behind* the structure of philosophy and health enunciated by the ancient manuscripts, I hope to validate the thesis that the arts empower, suture and heal both the body and the mind. Also, that both the process and the product, however intangible, are the same in all the arts.

Traditional Indian conception of the arts

Let us start by looking at how the ancients spelt out the goal of creative activity. They believed it to enable the creator to experience *ananda*, joy, and then to communicate it to the larger community, *Samaj*. This individual–community link is clearly prescribed as a part of the equation. This idea is not too far from the aim of modern and post-modern art – to please the creator first and only then the viewer. The traditional view also equates the notion of the sacred or the holy with the arts. From music, dance, painting, sculpture, theatre to literature, Indian culture enjoins upon all the arts the status enjoyed by a revealed scripture. This perspective has historically given the arts in India a status that is denied to them in many other major cultures.

Whatever the category, whether classical, folk or modern artistic pursuits, tradition, practice and now even science corroborate that the arts are completely therapeutic in nature (Gupta, 2005; Mamtani and Mamtani, 2005). Behind the apparent good health, longevity and incredible stamina of most dancers, musicians and visual artists lies the fact that the very nature of the work they do, i.e. sing, dance, paint, sculpt and write, in short create a work of art, is an endless source of pumping of metaphorical as well as actual iron, vitamins and nutrients into the body.

Before taking up each art individually and putting it under the lens of our investigation, it is necessary to reiterate their common antecedents, goals and structure. Awareness of the interrelationship of all existence, promoted not merely through religion, but also through life cycle patterns and the ancient Hindu belief that every atom of the universe is connected – in tune with quantum physics – colours artistic pursuit as well. As the sages say *Ekam Sat Vipra Bahudha Vadanti*: 'All that exists is one. The wise call it by many names' (Rig Veda 1.164.46).

This paradigm is illustrated by an apocryphal story from the *Vishnudharmottara Purana*, a 7th-century ad Sanskrit text. It recounts the tale of the king who desired to learn the art of painting. So he went to a master painter and asked to be taken on as his disciple. The master said he would do so but only after the king had learnt how to sculpt. The king sought out a teacher who would help him learn the art of sculpture. But the sculptor asked him to come back once he had learnt the art of dance. Once again the king set out in search of a guru, this time to help him learn dance. But when he found the right master, the latter asked him to first learn the arts of music and rhythm. Only after he had mastered all these arts could the king go back and learn how to paint.

This story points to the holistic underpinning of Indian art and aesthetics and to the linkages that each art form has with the other. Whether in the field of the performing arts such as music, dance, theatre or puppetry, visual arts such as painting and sculpture or the literary arts like classical novels and poetics, each form is inter-linked and suffused with an aesthetics derived from a common world view and a fairly similar approach to creativity. Below we shall look at each of the art forms from the perspective of traditional Indian teachings. Because even though they are all interconnected and inform each other, the various art forms have their own unique aspects.

Visual arts

The *Chitrasutra* of the *Vishnudharmottara Purana*, arguably the world's oldest treatise on art, not only provides a detailed account of the various schools, techniques and ideals of Indian painting, but specifies the aim of painting as one of communicating an emotion and causing particular spiritual states of mind. It says: 'Painting cleanses the mind and curbs anxiety, augments future good, causes the greatest delight, kills the evils of bad dreams and pleases the household deity.' Further, 'Painting is the best of all arts and is conducive to dharma (right conduct) and moksha (emancipation).' If its pictorial vision is a vivid, lively, refined, sophisticated, bold, vigorous and, of course, colourful combination of a love of naturalism and of decorating all kinds of surfaces and spaces, from a scroll painting to the walls of a hut, a chamber or temple altar, the impulse to adorn and ornament gets applied to mud, stone, metal, cloth, paper and even the human body, through applying paint, tattoos, henna and other herbal pastes and of course jewellery for each and every limb of the human frame.

It goes without saying that every detail of a traditional painting has some symbolic significance. Since the sacred was a prime impulse for taking the brush in hand, it required a high degree of internalization of the artist. The hundreds upon hundreds of illuminated texts that abound in the Buddhist art of India and Tibet, as well as the famous *thanka-s*, religious scroll paintings, were actually meant only for the initiated and the knowledgeable. This is clear from the following passage in the 'Hevajratantra', a medieval Buddhist text: 'If someone unworthy should see either book or painting, one will fail to gain perfection in this world or the next. To one of our tradition it may be shown any time' (Pal, 1984, p.19).

Music

The idea of music as therapy is a very old one in India. It is based on the precept of Nada Brahma, Sound is God. Almost all the great religions of the world talk about the Word that was there when the universe first appeared. While nobody is sure what this original word was, Sage Patanjali (between 650 ad and 850 ad), the founder of Yoga as a science, says that this first sound is a special Being and is expressed by the original word (Pranav). The veneration for music and those who create it is a continuing stream in Indian thought. Since Indian aesthetics and philosophy point to the arts as being akin to Yoga, it follows that their training and teaching, too, is in the nature of building blocks of Yogic discipline. The arts share with Yoga physical exercises, called Asanas, and specialized breathing techniques, the Pranayama.

In Indian classical music, as in deep meditation, the mind focuses on a single thought, here a note, for a long time. When contemplation (called Sanyam in Patanjali's works), reflection and concentration (samadhi) happen thus, they produces a sense of wellbeing and relaxation that stimulates or 'tickles' the pituitary gland and releases those chemicals into the body which produce a sense of pleasure. Though this process is not fully understood as yet, it is similar to what we feel when we hear soul-stirring music. It is known as the principle of equivalence. Different types of music, sung at different times of the day's time cycle and in different seasons, as enjoined by Hindustani music, stimulate feelings of sadness, anger, joy and peace.

Dance

Dance, worldwide, requires the presence of three elements: suppleness, strength and stamina. Indian dance also seeks to fulfil the criteria of making it enjoyable, providing an opportunity for self-expression, stimulating the whole body including at the cellular level, and challenging it to sharpen the development of a sound body and mind. An aspect which sets classical Indian dance apart from other major exercise systems, such as aerobics, is the requirement of symmetry and balance. In every classical style, whatever movement is done on the left is done on the right also. There is equal involvement of the arms and the legs. In each limb, every joint is involved. There is a rhythm and regularity in each set of movements. In just the opening piece of a traditional Bharat Natyam recital, the *Alarippu* (literally, the unfolding of petals), there is an amazing total of 238 movements, to be executed in just three minutes. They make the body bend, jump, stretch and leap as well as exercising the torso, the waist, the feet, the heels, the toes, the face and the neck.

Similarly, the use of the hands and the *mudras*, the technical word for hand gestures, common to all Indian classical dance styles, is meant not only to look beautiful and convey thought and meaning but is also designed as a therapeutic tool, providing acupressure on those nerve endings which help with specific health problems. Pursuit of the arts develops both the brain and brawn, creating a sound mind in a sound body. Since all Indian dance styles are danced barefoot, with close contact with the ground, the well-known benefits of acupressure, achieved through a vast variety of steps, are also part of the healing process.

In the course of one simple phrase, such as 'KITA THAKA THA DINGINATHOM' of Bharatanatyam, the ear listens to the gait, the eye follows the hands, the mind correlates the hands and feet to work together with the eyes and through repetition and intense practice a synchronization of the body, the mind and the soul, the *atman*, is achieved which is truly phenomenal. It is for these reasons that Indian dancers enjoy exceptional health, fitness and a disease-free body.

Traditional Indian conception of health

There are so many systems of treating disease, but according to both Indian philosophy and Ayurveda, the Indian system of medicine, there is only one science of health. If we broadly divide the various systems of treatment of disease into external and internal, the traditional Indian approach, as with other old world cultures, has been a judicious mixture of the two, with the larger emphasis being on the internal route composed of cultivation of the mind and body through regularly prescribed activity (such as the arts). Ayurveda does depend on externals, like organic drugs and herbal formulations, but its core is the belief that prevention is better than cure. Indeed, it goes further to stress that prevention is the *only* cure.

Here we need to look at the nature of the body according to Ayurveda. It is also the point at which Indian tradition departs from Western models. Ayurveda takes a holistic approach to treatment that entails aligning and balancing the physical and mental components of an individual, thereby equating equilibrium with health (Mishra, Singh and Dagenais, 2001). It is necessary to remember that our body is continually undergoing change. Our stomach lining changes every five days, the skin every four weeks and our liver gets a complete overhaul every six weeks. After every 12 weeks major changes appear even in the skeletal structure. Now, a body that changes its entire physical structure and schemata as quickly and as thoroughly as we have observed here cannot possibly be reduced to mechanical deductions of the sort that the allopathic system of healing presupposes. Pop a pill, and are you sure it will have the same effect on the liver, the spleen, the lungs, the skin today as it did a week ago when the doctor prescribed it? Research demonstrates that this ancient medicine has a profound therapeutic effect (Patwardhan and Mashelkar, 2009; Patwardhan *et al.*, 2005).

Conclusion

Indian classical arts are built on the knowledge that the *sharira*, the Sanskrit word for body, is the link between the earth and the cosmos, between humanity and divinity, and that the cycle of matter is forever revolving, forever dying, forever creating a new physical body. It is this constant replacement of matter, this continual re-creation, that, if it is to be helped to remain healthy, must be directed on the path of the creative impulse and to find its expression through the arts. This leads to the fundamental premise that true health needs to be created from within the body and with the help of awareness of its real nature. This is where the creative process comes in, particularly the role of the arts. Indian arts and culture traditionally reflect and uphold the view, across the many creative disciplines, that pursuit of the arts develops both brain and brawn, creating a sound mind in a sound body.

References

Gupta, B.S. (2005) 'Psychophysiological responsivity to Indian instrumental music.' *Psychology of Music 33*, 4, 363–372.

Mamtani, R. and Mamtani, R. (2005) 'Ayurveda and yoga in cardiovascular diseases.' *Cardiology in Review 13*, 3, 155–162.

Mishra, L., Singh, B.B. and Dagenais, S. (2001) 'Ayurveda: A historical perspective and principles of the traditional healthcare system in India.' *Alternative Therapies in Health and Medicine 7*, 2, 36–42.

Pal, P. (1984) *Tibetan Paintings*. London: Sotheby.

Patwardhan, B. and Mashelkar, R.A. (2009) 'Traditional medicine-inspired approaches to drug discovery: Can Ayurveda show the way forward?' *Drug Discovery Today 14*, 15/16, 804–811.

Patwardhan, B., Warude, D., Pushpangadan, P. and Bhatt, N. (2005) 'Ayurveda and Traditional Chinese Medicine: A comparative approach.' *Evidence-Based Complementary and Alternative Medicine 2*, 4, 465–473.

Singh, S.S. (2001) *The Role of Healing in Asia's Traditional Arts (with Special Reference to India)*. Keynote address to the Fourth International Asian Pacific Performing Arts Network, Seoul, Korea.

Chapter 14

Reflecting on Materials and Process in Sichuan, China

Jordan S. Potash and Debra Kalmanowitz

In thinking about the place of art therapy in Asia generally and in China specifically, we have needed to be open to what we have been seeing and experiencing, while remaining true to the principles of art therapy. In addition to therapy, clinical practice, and interpersonal relationships, we have also needed to consider important aspects of art making. In this chapter, we will explore both Western and traditional Chinese assumptions on media and materials, with reference to how they affected art therapy during a training in Sichuan, China, following the 2008 earthquake.

Background

Located in southwest China and being one of the largest provinces, Sichuan has more than 15 ethnic minorities that are both representative and distinct from the rest of China. Each of these groups has its own charisma, ethnic style, traditions, and customs. Known for China's panda reserves and as a gateway to Tibet, the area received a great deal of attention when it was hit by a devastating earthquake in May 2008 (Figure 14.1). The epicenter in Wenchuan (northwestern part of the province) occurred in the area that is home to the Qiang, one of China's recognized ethnic minority groups. Although they have a distinct culture, animistic beliefs, and unique tradition of embroidery, they have also had close contact with the Han Chinese (majority group) for centuries, which has led to an exchange of ideas and language (Yin, 1994).

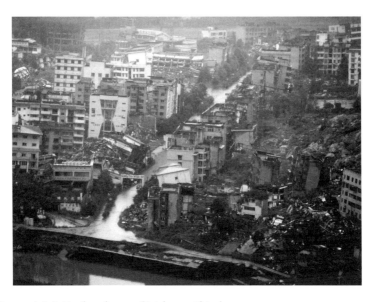

Figure 14.1 *Earthquake area (Beichuan, China)*

As part of the response effort, we were invited to join a team from Hong Kong to deliver an intensive training to provide teachers living and working in the area affected by the earthquake with basic skills in how to use art as a form of expression in their classroom. The training, titled "Using Arts as a Media for Healing: A Training Project for Sichuan School Teachers," was organized by the Centre on Behavioral Health at the University of Hong Kong, Beijing Tsing Hua University, and the Institute of Psychology, China Academy of Science, and sponsored by the Robert H.N. Ho Family Foundation Limited. It consisted of an initial three-day training and three supervision visits over the following year. The first day of the training included familiarization with the creative process and basics of trauma theory. The second day taught specific skills in the expressive arts. The third day offered teachers an opportunity to design an expressive arts activity and an expressive arts-based closing ritual. Rainbow Ho, a dance/movement therapist, delivered the module on the use of movement, while we facilitated a module on the use of visual arts modeled on the sensitive use of the art model (Kalmanowitz and Lloyd, 2005; Kalmanowitz and Potash, 2010). There were also accompanying staff to assist in research collection, program delivery, interpretation, and translation.

The training was arranged according to a train-the-trainer model and designed along the experiential learning model in order to give the teachers an experience of the expressive arts for non-educational pursuits. We thought it was important for the teachers to have an experience of art making and through this to begin to develop an intimate understanding of the creative process in order to apply it in their own unique settings. As trainers, we were aware that the approach we were taking was quite different to the style of education in China, which is typically more didactic and regimented. As expected, some of the participants struggled with this training style, and yet despite this, at the end of the first day, one of the participants, a doctor, addressed the group at large, stating:

> I know our education system is influenced by Confucius; we believe in the teacher being at the top… But maybe it is time to change… You [the teachers] are a light for your children— here you need to lead them by listening—because they want to be led.

The structure we created in Hong Kong before we left for Sichuan was a starting point, but we knew we would have to be open to adjusting it, according to what we found, while maintaining the principles that were important in using the arts to help children.

Assumptions on materials and process

When we review the history of Western art, we are reminded of the importance of the personal stories of the artists as well as their social–cultural–historical context in understanding the meaning of the works. These diverse contexts affect the content of the art and the materials, technique, and styles used (Barrett, 2003). Western art has been influenced by Christianity and the Church as reflected in numerous paintings depicting scenes from the Bible and the history of the Church. Western art has also been influenced by politics, with rich patrons commissioning and paying for work, while dictating subject matter. The representation of a personal view is a relatively new focus, but the one with which we are most familiar with today (Davies *et al.*, 2004).

Traditional Chinese painting is not dissimilar in that it fits into a long and rich artistic tradition. In this tradition the relationship between the painter and Chinese philosophy was traditionally intertwined. (There is a close relationship between painters, their personality, and Chinese philosophy.) Fundamental to this philosophy is the emphasis on the mood and the spirit of the image, be it landscape, calligraphy, nature, or portrait, and on depicting humans as living in harmony with heaven and earth (Bonan, 1995). These attitudes towards art reflect different ways of viewing the world.

Art therapy as a discipline has been influenced by both art history and psychology. In addition, the materials that we use and process that we subscribe are also influenced by our context. The trends in contemporary art practice and art therapy have been noted by Moon (2010), who documented changing ideas on the types of materials offered and how they are used in art therapy, which we will explore further in this chapter.

With regards to our Sichuan training, we made several observations, some of which appeared to challenge Western ideas about materials and process in art therapy, while others seemed to reveal certain universal similarities in art therapy across cultural borders. We present them here as considerations in building an art therapy model that is accessible in China and throughout Asia.

Assumption on process: Art making is for personal emotional expression

Kramer's (1966) definition of quality in art therapy includes the importance of *evocative power* and *internal consistency* for emotional expression and personal meaning, respectively. This idea puts forward the assumption that for art to be successful in art therapy it must carry an emotional intent that can be communicated to a viewer. Although not a problem in certain settings, this idea comes with certain culturally bound values on what qualifies as expression. While her ideas may have constituted a foundational idea in the Western field of art therapy, there may be movement towards seeing art not as limited to personal expression, but as a reflection of group needs and cultural values (Moon, 2010). Furthermore, Skaife (2001) suggested that a true use of the creative process in service of healing is an emphasis on how art making reflects intersubjectivity, that is a reflection of the interpersonal relationships and group identity. Expanding the notion of *personal emotional expression* is necessary, given that it is not automatically the case in all cultures. With regards to Chinese culture, Chinese people may tend more towards limited emotional expression out of respect for group harmony, living within one's expected role, or to avoid extremes that can lead to illness (Bond, 1993; Woo, 2009).

On the first day of the training, after a dance/movement exercise, we introduced an art activity designed to give participants exposure to art making. Our initial request was to suggest that the participants imagine a piece of paper and imagine holding a pencil to draw a shape in the air. Following this relatively unthreatening activity, we asked that they make the same marks as they made in the air, but this time using art materials. Next we instructed them to experiment with specific marks, such as thick and thin lines, long and short, continuous and dotted. In response to a cautiousness we witnessed, we moved from making art individually to a suggestion of making art in a group. Where there had been hesitation to explore individually, in groups the dynamic changed almost immediately. The group work seemed to free the participants from the incapacitating expectations of their own drawings.

On the last day of the training, a large mandala pre-cut into five pieces (Figures 14.2 and 14.3) was placed in the center of the room. Working in groups of ten, they used a range of drawing materials to create images of what they would take away from the training. After the pieces were brought back together, the dance and movement therapist led a movement activity around the mandala to allow participants to view it from all angles and to end the training.

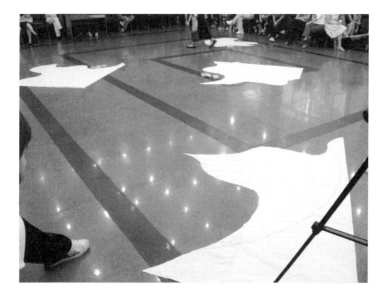

Figure 14.2 *Puzzle pieces*

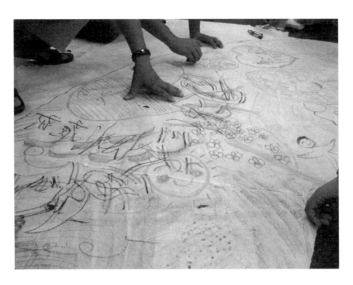

Figure 14.3 *Creating the puzzle pieces*

The responses to the different group activities possibly points to the difference between individual and collective art making. Whereas there was some hesitation or inability to engage the arts for exploration individually, when in groups the dynamic immediately changed. Quiet, trepidation, inhibition, and suspicion were replaced with laughter, animation, and experimentation. It's difficult to say definitively whether the activities up to that point served as a warm-up or if they were simply the group process. Later processing with the group and debriefing with fellow trainers let us know that the group activity seemed to allow the participants to feel that they were part of a larger whole; this in itself gave meaning to the activities.

From this observation, it would be easy to conclude that art making should have been offered as a collective experience in order to highlight the intersubjectivity. Gearing activities towards the group might ignore what occurred for individuals. Although throughout the training we were met with hesitation at the beginning of each activity, once engaged many of the participants seemed to become increasingly interested in experimenting with the materials. The participants seemed to benefit from the experiential learning, as we witnessed in some a sense of achievement, relaxation, enjoyment, an increased awareness on likes and dislikes, and willingness to take risks. Some comments from the participants in this regard were:

If you are willing to open up and work—then you can learn…
Willingness to try is important.

I am a person with low self-esteem. Today I was able to open
up and have confidence in my work.

My emotions became more and more stable in the process… I
became more self-assured through the stations.

I found my own experience drawing. I was not at all familiar
with clay, so I felt relaxed and free. I found that I had a bit of
artistic potential.

This type of learning could be transferred to their students based on one
teacher's comments on how exploring the materials helped her to see
"how we can help our students to choose" what materials are best or most
needed at a given time. Processing the art helped to give the experience
order and make connections between the experience, theory, and what
can be used in the classroom. Rather than conclude that either group or
individual activity is superior, this training highlighted the benefit from
both, despite the expected cultural norms.

Assumption on materials: Art materials have inherent emotional qualities

Another precept of art therapy is that various art materials have the ability
to affect emotional expression based on how their physical qualities
affect the ease of expression (Malchiodi, 2002; Rubin, 1984). Kagin and
Lusebrink (1978) put forward the idea of a continuum of expression based
on two interdependent factors related to the amount of energy it takes to
manipulate the material and emotional needs related to either catharsis
or understanding. All of the theories on the relationship between media
and emotions base their ideas on the objective, physical qualities of the
materials themselves, but suggest that these properties have the ability to
affect emotional expression.

While materials may not change across cultures, their use and
particularly the cultural rules that govern their use can vary drastically.
Even within Western culture, art history shows the dramatic ways in which
painting has changed from monochromatic cave paintings to realistic
narratives to surreal images and abstract expression. While these changes
have occurred over hundreds of years in the West, China's art traditions
have only gone through dramatic changes in the last several decades. As

one of the oldest continuous artistic traditions in the world, the earliest Chinese paintings were ornamental, consisting of patterns or designs, but also incorporated representations of the world. Despite the subject matter, traditional Chinese painting emphasizes the skillful application of the technique and careful application of the material. Artists used a brush to apply black or colored ink on paper or on silk, and their brushstrokes were seen as expressions of the spirit (Bonan, 1995).

The second day of the training was divided into a morning session on art materials and an afternoon session on structure and themes. In the materials session, participants came into the room, which was arranged in five stations with locally bought materials. The stations were collage, pencil on two different sizes of paper, markers on regular-size paper, paint, and clay. Participants spent 15–20 minutes at each station before moving to the next at the scheduled time. They were not given specific instructions, but were told to explore with the materials. Before switching to the next station, participants wrote reflection notes. After the participants had experimented with all the available materials, we gathered as a group to discuss their experience and emotional reactions, and how these may impact the use of art with their students. The debriefing from the art materials activity revealed several interesting themes. The experience led to a discovery of likes and dislikes, curiosity, and different levels of comfort with the materials.

Many participants enjoyed the collage station, describing it as "aimless" and "comforting." They found it helpful that the materials themselves provided some ideas for how to use them and what kind of images to create. They also found this the easiest material to use for those without prior skill or expertise in art making. Many participants commented on the metaphor of the process of being able to "discover new" and create something good from that which would otherwise be discarded.

Several participants agreed that drawing with pencil was challenging and uncomfortable. For some the small paper was restrictive, while for others the large paper was threatening. They did not like the limit of color or how the material could be used. Still, there was recognition that pencil was smooth and produced a solid image. In contrast, markers were favored due to the intensity and choice of color. They were seen as leading to more "beautiful" drawings. In comparison with other materials, participants commented on the permanency of the marks and the lack of ability to change them.

Of the materials that we offered, participants were the most familiar with painting. They described it as fluid and freeing, but also difficult to control. This awareness seemed to be both an advantage and impediment. Some participants described the ease with which they could mix colors and create images, whereas others felt it challenging. There seemed to be a discrepancy between the description of paint as liberating and the images that were created. These were generally confined to more traditional themes than those created using the other art materials.

Although it was unfamiliar to several participants, clay was seen as relaxing. Even those who were anxious at first found it soothing and enjoyable. The tactile experience and the unlimited changeability was described as having the ability to release negative emotions.

Those familiar with the theories on the expressive quality of art materials will most likely not be surprised by the way the teachers described their experience with the various materials. This lends some credibility to the possible universal expectations and inherent expressive characteristics of art materials. In fact, the similarity in responses is even more amazing given that many of the teachers came from a culture and lived in ways that would be considered incredibly foreign by Western practitioners and originators of these theories.

One notable difference was in painting. As previously mentioned, the images that emerged were not spontaneous expressions, but were restricted to themes traditional for Chinese painting. Most paintings were reminiscent of traditional Chinese landscapes: pictures of bamboo, blossoms, lotus flowers, or animals on a traditionally empty background (Figure 14.4). It's possible that this came about due to the types of paints used that resembled traditional ink. We offered this paint, as this is what was available locally, but we wonder if the paintings that emerged and the use of paint would have been different had we been able to offer acrylics or tempera paint.

What was especially interesting to us was that the material that was the most free seemed to come with cultural values that imposed the most control over how to use it. This dichotomy is interesting, because the Western idea of painting as emotional expression stands in contrast to the Chinese idea of ink on paper as the epitomy of sensitivity of expression. Even if we consider that a seemingly black and white painting consists of multiple shades of black and numerous brushstrokes, the mere mark on the paper is an expression of a feeling and spirit. This form of expression is certainly a different way to look at emotions than we do in the West. In the West our emotions are made explicit, given color and shape; expressing ourselves alludes to letting go, while expressing oneself through Chinese culture seems to allude to the exact opposite. Instead there is an encouragement to remain completely in the present and create the most sensitive mark possible by unifying body, mind, and spirit.

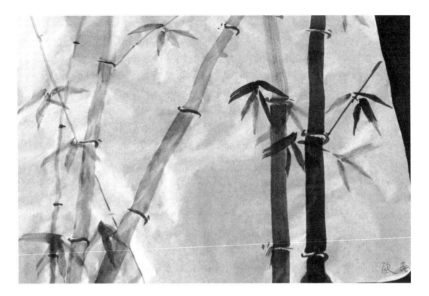

Figure 14.4 *Painting of bamboo*

What we observed was a divide between how the material was experienced and how it was actually applied. Having the emotional understanding that it was and could be freeing was limited by the cultural expectation of how it should have been used. This important observation speaks to a gap in Western art therapy ideas, such as those postulated by Kagin and Lusebrink (1978). Their description of the integrative Creative Level frequently refers to the interaction of the individual with the media, but does not seem to specifically take into account cultural variance. Given that they highlight the ultimate goal of unification of media and intent to bring forward a state of fulfillment in the artist, we may need to consider how individuals accommodate the media within their own cultural reference.

Assumption on form: Traditional and decorative arts are not personally expressive

Art exists in every culture; it is used for healing, ritual, and decoration and provides meaning to life experiences (Dissanayake, 1995). As previously stated, the emphasis on the personal experience of art making in the West, and particularly in art therapy, implies the primacy of individual expression. It is essential to know how art functions in a given society in order to understand how these factors inform art created in art therapy. Moon (2010) points out that art therapists can begin to follow contemporary artistic traditions by finding a place for crafts in art therapy without seeing them as lesser than objects of expression. Redefining indications of quality can be determined by adherence to tradition, and the emphasis can be on the interaction with the material. Even embodied in the seemingly repetitive patterns of traditional arts, there are embedded sparks of creativity and expression in terms of choice of subject matter or process of creation. As an example, the Qiang people are long known for their handicraft, embroidery, and carpet weaving, which date back to the Ming dynasty in the 14th century. In fact this minority group use all the arts to make meaning in their lives; they create folk stories and use dance and music to express their individual and collective challenges (Yin, 1994).

In an attempt to demonstrate the role of structure and provide some support to the teachers who survived the earthquake, in the afternoon of the second day we provided clear directions for an activity. After much discussion and debate between us on the nature of the directive, we asked the teachers to create art about their professional strengths and a challenge they had been experiencing in the classroom since the earthquake. The comfort with art making that they had been developing up to that point seemed to come to an end. Asking participants to directly focus on their feelings within a Western way of working seemed to largely result in an inability to move forward in the process. The art that was created felt forced and required a great deal of prompting and support from us and the other facilitators.

In considering the culturally accepted art forms and looking at what occurred throughout the morning media exploration, we wonder how we could have presented this theme differently, if at all. Up until this point in the training, the focus had been on gaining comfort with materials and using them to create spontaneous forms. By offering the directive in the way that we did, the focus of the ensuing activity became about individual emotional expression. Our directive, although well meaning and sensitively placed, should have taken into account the possible need to offer a structured *form* in which to convey a story.

Speaking to the teachers about their experiences of art, reflecting on the images produced at the morning painting station, and walking through the stalls of crafts dealers revealed that art is used for multiple purposes, almost none of which relate to personal emotional expression. Rather, we saw specific images—such as landscapes, day-to-day life, and celebrations—depicted over and over again, in addition to intricate designs and patterns. The creators take great pride in them, but there may be little or no trace of the individual artist. Still, each image tells a story and conveys an essential idea or value.

An important question for art therapists to consider is what happens when art is not perceived as emotionally expressive, but as a form of decoration, a re-creation of nature, or a form of meditation. Another question is finding a place in art therapy for art that strives to express the very essence or spirit of an experience. The essence of a mountain, for example, may be painted, so that, the artist not only conveys the physical mountain in traditional forms, but also the way in which the artist sees and understands this mountain. The focus shifts from one's private emotional response to conveying the dynamic aspects of the experience in the personal, transpersonal, historical and cultural context

It seems that it is too simplistic to say that the traditional arts in Sichuan do not reflect an emotionally expressive nature. As we have seen, they seem to reflect collective ideas, rather than personal ones. Since the training, we have begun to wonder how to use the imagery from the traditional arts as an entry point to expression within traditionally accepted and known images. For example, in the future we could discuss how a landscape painting captures a moment that is not immediately present, may no longer exist, or is offered as an ideal. From this starting point, we may be able to begin a discussion of how to record or capture what is not present or unseen. We may then be able to transition into examples of seasonal landscapes as to how they reflect and affect emotions. In addition to landscape paintings, other traditional images related to community celebrations or daily activities may have provided other channels for story telling on strengths, challenges, and feelings. Bringing together all of these ideas may have supported the teachers by grounding them in known art forms, which in turn may have allowed them the possibility of capturing special moments in the life of the community or individual.

Conclusion

This chapter is limited by our observation over this short time with the participants and, as such, we acknowledge that our reflections should be considered in this light. Still, the observations we made and questions we raised point to differences in how to use and offer materials within specific cultural contexts. Some artists like to represent the world as they see it, by working towards a naturalistic imitation of an object or scene, creating the illusion of perspective and space, while others may work on showing the inner spirit, emotions, or feelings of the individuals and the paintings, expressing the artist's intention. It has been important to us to unravel our preconceptions and assumptions, in an attempt to understand our experience in light of our art therapy training. The intersection of what constitutes expression, what role media have on art making, and the place of structure are entwined in all art-making experiences. By looking at tenets of art therapy theory through multiple cultural lenses, we hoped to have demonstrated culturally sensitive and informed ways of working.

References

Barrett, T. (2003) *Interpreting Art: Reflecting, Wondering, and Responding.* Boston: McGraw-Hill.

Bonan, G. (1995) *Gate to Chinese Calligraphy.* Beijing, China: Foreign Languages Press.

Bond, M.H. (1993) "Emotions and their expression in Chinese culture." *Journal of Nonverbal Behavior 17*, 4, 245–262.

Davies, J., Denny, W., Hofrichter, F., Jacobs, J., Roberts, A. and Simon, D. (2004) *Janson's History of Art: The Western Tradition,* 7th edn. Upper Saddle River, NJ: Pearson Prentice Hall.

Dissanayake, E. (1995) *Homo Aestheticus: Where Art Comes from and Why.* Seattle: University of Washington Press.

Kagin, S.L. and Lusebrink, V. (1978) "The expressive therapies continuum." *Art Psychotherapy 5*, 4, 171–179.

Kalmanowitz, D. and Lloyd, B. (2005) *Art Therapy and Political Violence: With Art Without Illusion.* London: Routledge.

Kalmanowitz, D. and Potash, J.S. (2010) "Ethical considerations in the global teaching and promotion of art therapy to non-art therapists." *Arts in Psychotherapy 37*, 20–26.

Kramer, E. (1966) "The Problem of Quality in Art." In: E. Ulman and P. Dachinger (eds) *Art Therapy in Theory and Practice* (pp.43–59). Chicago: Magnolia Street.

Malchiodi, C. (2002) *The Soul's Palette: Drawing on Art's Transformative Powers for Health and Well-Being.* Boston and London: Shambhala.

Moon, C.H. (ed.) (2010) *Materials and Media in Art Therapy: Critical Understandings of Diverse Artistic Vocabularies.* New York, NY: Routledge.

Rubin, J.A. (1984) *The Art of Art Therapy.* New York, NY: Brunner/Mazel.

Skaife, S. (2001) "Making visible: Art therapy and intersubjectivity." *International Journal of Art Therapy 6*, 2, 40–50.

Woo, T.T. (2009) "Emotions and self-cultivation in *Nü Lunyu* (Woman's Analects)." *Journal of Chinese Philosophy 36*, 2, 334–347.

Yin, M. (1994) *China's Minority Nationalities.* Beijing, China: Foreign Languages Press.

Chapter 15

The Integration of Arts Therapy and Traditional Cambodian Arts and Rituals in Recovery from Political-Societal Trauma

Carrie Herbert

All people share the gift of imagination, for creativity is not restricted to a chosen meritorious few. Ascendant personalities who survived the Cambodian trauma with the force of will and the strength to dream their dreams of hope demonstrate that Cambodian culture is endowed with unlimited human potential to use the inner world of imagination to find new truths. (Bit, 1991, p.152)

In an arts therapy residential programme conducted by the Ragamuffin Project in 2004, over 50 leaders of community programmes met to consider the impact of Cambodia's past and present on the Cambodian people. Mapping out the history of Cambodia through image in a large painting on the floor, the group was asked to choose periods of history that they felt were the most significant in shaping Cambodia in the present. They chose the following:

- Angkorian (between 802 and 1220 ad when the Khmer civilization created the temples of Angkor and the arrival and impact of Indian sea merchants)

- United States' 'secret' bombing of Cambodia (1969–1973)

- Pol Pot, Khmer Rouge and the prolonged period of conflict (1979–1998)

The participants were divided into six different groups and each asked to select one of the periods of history. They then represented each period through a performance, storytelling, drama and/or music. In doing so, they identified what each period in history contributed to Cambodian society and what this would convey to future generations. Key themes seemed to repeat themselves from one period to the next: imagination, creativity and resilience; invasion, threat and violent conflict; religions, superstition and fear; and desecration and creation of cultural symbols of national and collective identity. The group discussed how throughout history there are cycles of creativity and destruction. In more recent history, and right up to the present day, pervasive fear, violence and conflict remained present and parallels were drawn from the past to the present. Looking forward, they expressed their desperate fear for the future of Cambodian young people and that history would repeat itself. The groups representing the present and future held the same despair and hopelessness as those in the times of war and conflict. The past was in the present and people had become stuck in the country's history.

The group identified the importance of metaphors and symbols that represented the strength of Cambodian identity. In exploring possible solutions for the present problems and finding hope for the future, it was the pre-Angkorian group whose creative voice danced throughout history, with wisdom sourced in the natural world and the images and metaphors of nature. These were the cycles of life from birth to death and re-birth, the importance and symbolism of animals and the need for balance and harmony between all things. In their drama they became animals, trees and Cambodian people. They improvised and sang 'to sing and dance in harmony with nature, to create, imagine and believe'. The Angkorian group identified the importance of man-made symbols that represented the strength of Cambodian identity such as the Apsara, the temples of Angkor Wat and the four faces of Buddha. The group then continued to sing a contemporary pop song about the temples and then *Nokor Reach* (Chuon, 1941) the national anthem that is based on a Cambodian folk tune, reinstated after the war in 1993. It speaks of Cambodia's ancient spiritual essence found in Kings throughout the ages, and the eternal identity of the Khmer symbolized by the temples of Angkor Wat:

> Heaven protects our King and gives
> him happiness and glory so to
> reign over our souls and our destinies.
> The one being, heir of the

Sovereign Builders, guiding the proud old Kingdom.
Temples are asleep in the forest, Remembering
the splendour of Moha
Nokor. Like a rock the Khmer race is
eternal. Let us trust in the fate
of Kampuchea, the empire which challenges the ages.
Songs rise up from the pagodas to the glory of holy Buddhist
faith. Let us be faithful to our ancestors'
belief. Thus heaven will
lavish its bounty towards the ancient
Khmer country, the Moha Nokor.

The image of Angkor Wat is a powerful national symbol that adorns the Cambodian flag and often emerges in creative arts therapy sessions when exploring an empowered self-image or collective identity. Bit (1991) challenges Cambodians to summon the strength to liberate themselves from what he describes as 'the war ambience' (p.153). He goes on to suggest how the long history of enforced helplessness has psychologically conditioned Cambodians to live with fear as an ever-present feature of their lives. His concluding plea is:

We need desperately to cultivate new creativities, which can make Cambodia a safe and moral society, instead of a desperate collection of warlord gangs moving from crisis to crisis and ultimately to self-destruction. Imagination and a spiritual awakening is needed. (p.156)

This chapter explores how the imagination and creativity through the traditional arts, ritual and the emergence of creative arts therapy is restoring resilience, esteem and identity for Cambodians in their recovery from political-societal trauma.

Power of the arts and cultural symbols in the survival and restoration of identity

Cambodia is thirsty for the power of imagination – the healing effect, which only works of art can provide... (Amrita Performing Arts, 2009, para.1)

It is estimated that 70 per cent of the current Cambodian population is under the age of 30 years old (Mydans, 2009). Chakryia Phal, a 30-year-old Cambodian-American art therapist who has recently moved back to Cambodia, reflected on how children in Cambodia seem to immerse themselves in Western and Asian pop culture. She also noted how young people in more developed areas of the nation, such as Phnom Penh, are emulating the hairstyles, clothing and makeup of Korean pop singers. Every night, at the Olympic stadium in Phnom Penh, dance classes are held and teenagers line up to learn how to pop their hips out and move their body to the beat of modern music, while the older generation are still doing aerobics to the beat of Khmer classics (personal communication, 30 April 2011).

Chakryia noted that the traumatized children she works with have shown little interest in exploring the traditional arts. They live in Phnom Penh, a city that is evolving and constantly changing. It is as though the city is trying to find its identity, and so it is constantly shedding its skin. The children are the same. It is not that there is a complete rejection of Khmer culture; but that they embrace the Khmer culture of now and not one of their parents. The socio norms and rules of their parents' time are seen as being too traditional, too strict and too primitive. It is not uncommon to hear kids say *boran* (old fashioned) as a sneer forms on the corner of their lips. Things that are seen as boran or traditional, such as playing traditional instruments, classical dance and the traditional arts, are associated with their parents' generation and dismissed. Phal asked, 'I wonder what the impact of them not exploring traditional arts and culture is?' Commenting on this observation, another arts therapist, Panchakna Khlok, noted:

> I see this creating enormous tension and conflict in families, and it may impact on their ability to find their Cambodian identity and how the history of the previous generation affects them today. (Personal communication, 2 May 2011)

In contrast to this observation from the city, Chakryia added, 'I find that children living in the countryside are still interested in traditional arts. There's still a sense of pride and national identity' (personal communication, 2 May 2011).

A classical Cambodian dancer (Pasles, 2000) explained that the Khmer Rouge killed between 80 and 90 per cent of artists, musicians and dancers in the country with only a handful surviving. After the Khmer Rouge years, artists and Cambodian arts have slowly been redeemed, thereby reviving traditions. Traditional Khmer dance has been one of Cambodia's national symbols since Angkorian times. Working with refugees from Vietnam and Cambodia in Indonesia, Shapiro (as cited in Pasles, 2000) witnessed how dance was the most important element in surviving violence and loss. Phim (as cited in Pasles, 2000) echoed this observation, explaining:

> To be a Cambodian dancer, you do not feel you are only a dance. You feel like you carry a very important part of Cambodian culture in you. It's a way of connecting the present to the past, the people to their ancestors. (Pasles, 2000, para.21)

Reinvigorating symbols

Cultural symbols live in the imagination. Jung (1964) talked about how unification with symbols of the anima and animus link us to the divine or true self. Wherever he looked across cultures, he found the same archetypes and thus came to conceptualize them as fundamental forces that exist beyond us. He found their representation in ancient myths as elemental spirits and Jung sought to connect with this deep and ancient experience. Historically in Cambodia, the Apsara (Figure 15.1) is seen in Khmer culture as a messenger of the divine.

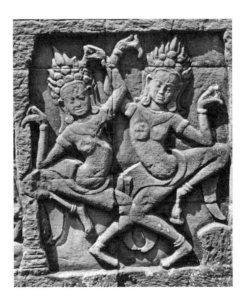

Figure 15.1 *Apsara*

According to Shapiro-Phim (2005):

> The Apsara, in her golden jewelry and glistening brocade, has come to be a symbol of Cambodia, and an emblem of the country's mythical-historical past. Carved in the thousands, images of celestial women line the walls of the country's ancient temple in the Angkor region, and are seen as links between humankind and the heavens. In one Cambodian myth an Apsara pairs with a sage, and through this union the Khmer people come into being. (p.5)

The Apsara dancer is a powerful collective symbol for women in Cambodia. Panchakna Khlok worked with an 11-year-old girl with Down syndrome who was trafficked and suffered terrible sexual abuse. She has difficulty verbally communicating her needs and is often misunderstood and dismissed by others who see her as different, ugly and strange. Khlock explained:

> I asked her to draw a picture of how she was feeling. No words came. She scribbled like a tiny child and then spontaneously began to make movements and gestures. She started dancing like an Apsara, her fingers flexing backwards, her body was full of beauty, poise and grace. Her smile was wide and it was the first time I had seen her find a sense of joy and peace. It was as if her spirit had risen above all her suffering inside. (Personal communication, 2 May 2011)

When brought into consciousness through embodiment, the Apsara can dignify the soul of a girl or woman whose life has been shattered and where words and language simply cannot suffice. The Apsara, as symbol of the divine and union with the soul of a person, often emerges in creative arts therapy work in Cambodia.

Panna (a pseudonym) is a 30-year-old woman who attends creative arts therapy supervision with me at Ragamuffin's Arts Therapy Centre in Phnom Penh. She works with traumatized children and contacted me in a crisis, explaining:

> I don't know what is wrong with me. I am angry and reacting to everyone and everything. It is violent and I am causing many problems for people around me. I feel like my self is split into pieces. I cannot find the earth beneath my feet, I feel like I am going crazy.

Using guided meditation I asked her to imagine an image of the person she fears is going crazy. Opening her eyes she describes a girl with flames coming out of her head, her face contorted and angry. After drawing the image from her imagination onto a big piece of paper, Panna laughed and commented, 'See, she is crazy, this is why everyone hates her!'

I suggested the girl might have some important things to tell us and maybe to those who think she is crazy. Panna named her Ame and, through dialoguing with the image, Ame found her voice and began to tell her story:

> I am 18 years old and my life is surrounded by violence, my father drinks and beats my mother every day. It's awful and frightening; nowhere is safe. My brother has turned to using drugs and is involved in a gang, and they go out at night and I know they do bad things. Sometimes they are violent too, just to get more drugs, more money, and then more drugs; I'm scared of them. All the neighbours around us hate us, they want us to leave, but they are doing violent things too; I saw them beat their children. Maybe there is violence everywhere; I feel it is my fault. I didn't place the fire in the right place in the house; this is why all these bad things happen to us.

We discovered that Ame believes that she was the cause of these problems. Her mother and grandmother told her that she made the fire in the wrong part of the home, so everything was doomed. The belief served to justify the family's violence and destruction, and Ame was held responsible.

Panna explained that the girl represented her and that this was the true story of her life. Giving voice to her story, Panna realized she had locked so much rage within her in the past that it was now lashing out uncontrollably in the present. Through movement, voice and drum, we explored how the anger of her childhood could be expressed. Panna's energy moved from a place of fear to a place of powerful energy. Following and supporting her expression, I used a drum to mirror her and reflect back her energy to assure her that she was heard. Panna laughed and said, 'I feel like I want to dance.' She began to dance as if she was the fire around the room, furious, wild, spontaneous and free.

At the end of the session, I returned to guided visualization to help her ground her energy. I asked, 'What image comes into your body and imagination now?' Panna opened her eyes and said, 'I see an Apsara dancer.' When asked to demonstrate, she stood on one leg with her foot flexed to the sky and her arms and hands unfolded in the gesture of an

Apsara dancer (Figure 15.2). She exclaimed, 'I feel balance and strength even on one leg! It's like the Khmer proverb that describes an Apsara as soft and strong. The Apsara is an angel, she is spirit; maybe she is my true spirit.' For Panna this session was a breakthrough from beliefs that had held her hostage to her fears and had caused her to act out with the same degree of violence that she had endured. The symbol became a transformational bridge to her rediscovering an aspect of herself that had become lost to her and was her ultimate source of dignity and power.

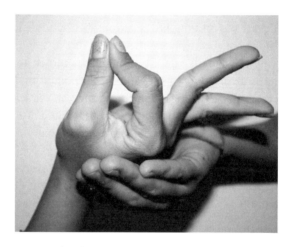

Figure 15.2 *Apsara hand gesture*

Recreating rituals for grief

Dara (pseudonym) lost both her child and husband during the Pol Pot time; she had tried to kill herself with poison a number of times, but had been rescued by her neighbours. She was depressed and suffered panic attacks and nightmares. Dara recognized she had not wanted to live since this time; she felt ashamed to be alive. She told the story of her 11-year-old daughter becoming sick and how the Pol Pot soldiers wouldn't let her take her to get medical care; they took her themselves. Dara never saw her again. Dara remembers running through the forest in the dark to try and find her; she returned a day later broken hearted to find her husband had also been taken and killed. Her pain was intolerable and she was unable to say anything, otherwise she too would be killed; she kept silent. Inside, her heart shattered and she said that her soul had fled. Now remarried with a family again, Dara feels life has never returned; she feels like there are ghosts in and all around her. I asked her if she knew what the ghosts wanted to say. Dara looked away as if it was a strange question; she muttered, 'Everyone thinks I am mad!' Then she suddenly said, 'The ghosts need to have their say and then they can go.' Dara was surprised, and for a moment her head lifted and she glanced at me. As we talked further Dara said, 'Maybe they are my husband, daughter and me still lost in the forest.' She cried out loud, 'I couldn't help them; I couldn't find them. I never buried their bodies to say goodbye.'

Over the next few sessions we talked and created together a ritual that Dara could use to let the ghosts speak and say goodbye. She drew pictures of her family, and placed white flowers on one of these. 'It's like a funeral for my family; my grandmother taught me to do this as a young girl when my aunt died,' she said. Before she came to the session Dara said she had gone to the temple to make an offering to free the spirits. Dara wanted to sing a song to say her final goodbye; it was a song from the Phleng Pinpeat tradition. This tradition accompanies funeral processions and is sad and sombre. Cambodians believe this music is a communication link between earth and the heavens (Ah Bee, 2011). Halfway through the song Dara broke down and wept. There was stillness and, after a long time, peace.

Rituals can be powerful cultural traditions full of the arts, meaning and symbols. Speaking of the power of ritual, McNiff (1998) writes, 'When art and psychotherapy are joined, the scope and depth of each can be expanded, and when working together, they are tied to the continuities of humanity's history of healing' (p.259). Dara created a ritual for an event that could never have taken place at the time. I enabled her to acknowledge her profound pain, and to grieve. As a therapist, taking part in this process enabled me to be a part of this world, one where to have only spoken about it would have reduced its meaning and interrupted the flow of mourning. Krause (1998) describes how ritual is the work of art.

Reclaiming lost traditions

Mango Tree Garden (Mango Tree Garden, n.d.) is a community-based programme. The programme has a holistic and child-centred approach. The children are respected and honoured, as is childhood and the natural, cultural and spiritual surroundings in which they live. Childhood is celebrated through creative play that is sensitive to the local culture. Creativity is a means for children to discover their own strengths and originality as they draw from their cultural, natural and spiritual resources to heal emotional and spiritual wounds.

I was invited by the Mango Tree Garden community play project to provide some workshops for the elders and leaders of the community where they were developing a therapeutic play programme. Sok, a man in his 70s, his carved skin testimony to the years of life experience, hung his head heavy with despair. Sok has lived through war and conflict, poverty and hardship and is currently one of the village elders in a provincial area outside Phnom Penh. When we met with Sok to explore how the elders could effectively support the children in the community who experience high levels of poverty, violence and child labour, he was sitting with two women elders and three monks.

We began the meeting with meditation. The monks led us in a chant, a blessing for our time together. There was an atmosphere of timelessness. Once we had finished, I asked them to teach us one of the games they played with the children. The game they chose was a game of the mother hen with her chicks. It is a Cambodian game about mothering, protection and invasion. The mother hen must protect a line of chicks behind her from an eagle who is trying to steal the chicks. As we played there was much laughter, and a fierce protectiveness as everyone took it in turns to be the mother hen. After the game we talked about their role in the community of protecting the children and the challenge of this. The play facilitated a discussion of how they felt about the level of violence in the community, the impact on the children and how they feared for their children's future. They talked about the distress of the mother hen and how this reminded them all of the war and being under attack and threat. In being the chicks they identified with the children in the community and their vulnerability, and also with their own childhoods.

Sok explained that they did not play much as children; they had to work hard and, when the war came, play had to become invisible. If the children were seen to play they would be scolded. The parents were so afraid to get caught, because if they were, terrible things would happen to them and their children.

I suggested to Sok that he close his eyes and see what he saw in his mind. I then asked him to draw what he saw. He exclaimed, 'I have never in all my life drawn anything.' After a while, however, he opened his eyes and tentatively drew with a blue crayon. He drew a picture of a flute, a Khmer traditional instrument. I asked if it sang and he laughed, 'No, it's a flute, just a flute.' Together we began to wonder what sound it might make. We then stopped for lunch and came back together in the afternoon. Sok appeared, late, apologizing, full of energy with a bundle of papers in his hands. These sheets were filled with sketches of traditional instruments. Sok had drawn a whole orchestra. 'I remember them and I knew how to play them all.' Sok began to tell the group the story of being a wedding singer when he was a young man: 'I would get invited to sing at weddings, play instruments and teach others.' I asked him if he could remember a wedding song. There was silence as the group waited expectantly. His voice broke out, trembling at first and then strong and clear across the countryside around us. There were tears in everyone's eyes. He sang a blessing song, sung whilst parents tie red string around the bride and groom's wrists.

Sok began to weep. He spoke of how he had lost his parents in the war, and how worried he was about the future of his children and community and the loss of tradition. We talked about the role he could still have: 'Maybe I can teach the children to play these instruments and sing.' This was in 2002; today in the heart of his community a local non-governmental organization (NGO), Mango Tree Garden, is flourishing, set in the heart of the pagoda. Where Sok sat is a playground, and a team of dedicated volunteers run weekly therapeutic play activities involving storytelling, songs, the visual arts, music and drama.

Conclusion

In art shops and galleries in Cambodia, you will find jewellery and works of art created from the metal of disarmed landmines as a testament to how trauma can be transformed. Kites fly again on the skyline at dusk as crowds of people of all ages line up to dance together. Weddings and funerals are always to be found blocking one street or another across the city; there are carvings in stone and paintings hanging in galleries across the country. Oxen carts have come, at an oxen-led pace, to the city streets from the heart of the countryside, carrying a cargo of popular pottery crafts. Silk is brought to market from the silk island where artisans weave beautiful designs. There is also a circus and hip hop; visual artists exhibit in galleries and Cambodian traditional dancers and musicians now perform across the world – the traditional and contemporary arts in Cambodia are alive and diverse.

The traditional arts are an emblem of a country's national pride and, as such, symbols of empowerment and faith. The classical arts provide a reference for individual and collective cultural identity. They are rich in symbolism, wisdom and the portrayal of Cambodian beauty, dignity and strength. They play a key role in empowering Cambodian people, who suffered a loss of cultural dignity during and after the Khmer Rouge holocaust, to experience redemption through identification with their remarkable culture; a culture that pre-dates the Pol Pot regime and one that lies at the core of what it means to be Cambodian. At the Ragamuffin Project's Creative Arts Therapy Centre in the heart of Phnom Penh, dedicated young Cambodian art therapists work every day with children and young people whose lives have been shattered by trafficking, violence, abuse, AIDS and addictions. As these issues remain endemic in Cambodia, there is a growing generation using both traditional and free forms of creative expression to rediscover and reclaim a deep sense of themselves and their community. From their experiences of empowerment and healing, we can imagine the impact on every aspect of society if it were exposed to this creative healing force, as Cambodia moves from a period of destruction to one of recovery from political-societal trauma and future promise.

References

Ah Bee (2011) 'Khmer music – The three types of Phleng Khmer.' Available at www. EzineArticles.com/2971371, accessed on 4 November 2011.

Amrita Performing Arts (2009) *Current Projects: 3 Years, 8 Months, 20 Days and Breaking the Silence.* Available at http://amritaperformingarts.org/currentproject.asp, accessed on 8 March 2011.

Bit, S. (cd.) (1991) *The Warrior Heritage. A Psychological Perspective of Cambodian Trauma.* Le Cerrito, CA: Seanglim Bit.

Choun, N. (1941) Nokor Reach. Available at www.embassy.org/cambodia/anthem.html, accessed on 8 March 2011.

Jung, C.G. (1964) *Man and His Symbols.* New York, NY: Doubleday and Company.

Krause, I. (1998) *Therapy Across Culture.* London: Sage Publications.

Mango Tree Garden (2001) Available at www.mangotreegarden.org, accessed on 17 November, n.d.

McNiff, S. (1998) *Trust the Process: The Artist Guide to Letting Go.* Boston, MA: Shambhala.

Mydans, S. (2009) 'Pain of Khmer Rouge era lost on Cambodian youth.' *New York Times,* 8 April. Available at www.nytimes.com/2009/04/08/world/asia/08cambo.html, accessed on 4 November 2011.

Pasles, C. (2000) 'Dancing Through the Dark: Film-maker shows how core art form helped Cambodians deal with genocide.' *L.A. Times,* 15 February. Available at http:// articles.latimes.com/2000/feb/15/local/me-64612, accessed on 4 November 2011.

Shapiro-Phim, T. (2005) *Tradition and Innovation in Cambodian Dance – A Curriculum Unit for Post-Secondary Level Educators.* Available at http://seap.einaudi.cornell.edu/post-secondary_teaching_materials, accessed 11 January 2011.

PART 5

Models of Art Therapy

Chapter 16

Group Art Therapy in Japan

A Framework for Providing Cross-Cultural Art Activities with Psychiatric Adult Patients

Shinya Sezaki

The purpose of this chapter is to demonstrate how art therapists can successfully conduct group sessions for psychiatric adult patients in Japan. The adaptation of art therapy theories and techniques to Japanese patients are primary concerns for practitioners who have been trained in other countries. Sue and Sue (1990) argue that psychotherapies have been conceptualized in Western individualistic terms and "share certain common components of White culture in their values and beliefs" (p.30). In fact, Japanese people possess cultural values, social customs, and communicative styles which are different from Western norms. These factors are believed to have some level of influence on the procedures and outcomes of Western-style art therapy conducted for Japanese patients.

I completed my graduate study in art therapy and clinical training in the United States, and have been practicing in a Japanese psychiatric hospital for over ten years. My style of art therapy is eclectic; however, I often utilize the theme-oriented and structured approach to art therapy with Japanese patients. Previously, I explored interdisciplinary viewpoints of therapeutic goals (Sezaki and Bloomgarden, 2000), which are forerunners of "Multi-axial Art Therapy Goals for Patients" (Sezaki, 2007). These treatment goals, incorporated with the theme-oriented and structured approach, have enabled me to devise and conduct new art activities within the Japanese medical system. The following descriptions are my research and case studies about the framework for providing creative art activities in Japanese psychiatric settings.

Theme-oriented approach to group art therapy

The theme-oriented approach to group art therapy is a way of offering specific issues, themes, or directions to the group, suggested by the therapist or the group members. This approach has both benefits and flaws from an art therapist's viewpoint. Case and Dalley (1992) point out that the art therapist is able to offer suitable themes that allow the clients to understand the creative process in a fairly controlled way, but the group relationship is likely masked by the struggle to gain a favorable relationship with the therapist. Therefore, Case and Dalley maintain that the approach "may be suitable for short-stay clients who need to explore specific issues or for those not able to benefit from working with the anxiety that attends an analytically oriented group" (p.216).

There are a few good reasons why the theme-oriented approach to group art therapy is helpful in working with Japanese patients. Japanese people are usually not accustomed to expressing themselves freely. They tend to hesitate when drawing or painting because they believe they lack artistic skills, which makes them feel self-conscious. Liebmann (1986) contends that having a theme can help focus those people who have difficulty in creating a piece of art. Some patients prefer having a theme and taking part in activities like collage making—with themes such as "Collecting What I Like"—while others are quite creative and may require a less structured atmosphere in creating their artwork.

Another rationale for using a theme in group art therapy with Japanese patients is that the relationship between the therapist and patients is hierarchical in Japanese culture. Japanese society has historically been very hierarchical, with order and structure being highly respected. Many of these historical social constructs are still relevant in modern Japan today. For example, Morita therapy and Naikan are transpersonal and existential psychotherapies (Walsh, 1989) derived from Japanese Zen philosophy (Reynolds, 1989). They are highly structured and systematic therapeutic styles. Because some patients will be reluctant to freely express themselves, and because of the inherent respect for order and structure, it is important to consider that a non-directive approach may potentially lead to confusion.

The idea of conducting a theme-oriented group has been discussed in Japanese art therapy literature. Iwai, Horii and Ito (1985) proposed their theme-oriented approach to conducting group art therapy for patients with neurosis. They used three drawing themes: a tree, a landscape, and circles designed to represent the patient's family. They argued that these three themes manifested, respectively, the patient's state of ego, cognitive state of space gestalt, and relationship with their families. This approach has been used for other inpatient groups as well (Mine *et al.*, 1991). Iwai and his colleagues also developed the "Picture Explaining and Role Exchange Technique" for neurotic or psychosomatic patients. In this group technique, group members, including the therapist, turn over their completed pictures. Next, they introduce another member's picture to the group, while asking the other members how they feel about it. After this introduction, the pictures are returned to the original creator, and then he or she explains the piece again. It seems that Iwai and his colleagues thought that this technique would make their positions as therapists less directive and authoritarian as they recognized that strong leadership often prevents the patients from communicating with each other in group sessions.

Conducting a theme-oriented and structured group in Japan

Yalom (1983) stresses, "An externally imposed structure is the first step to a sense of internal structure" (p.108). Yalom's point is particularly valid in a Japanese social setting. Group structures often exert a sense of psychological protection and are helpful in reducing the patients' fear of disorder and chaos. A scheduled time and set procedures also provide a form of structure that allow Japanese patients to benefit from art therapy. Usually, sessions using this approach are 90 minutes long, and consist of several procedures. The following description is a working model for art therapists conducting Japanese group sessions.

Orientation (5 minutes)

To provide the Japanese patients with a sense of structure, and reduce their anxiety, the therapist communicates the purpose and guidelines of the therapy session at the beginning. Alternatively, the therapist can have one person in the group present the guidelines of therapy by providing a printed card. This task seems to enhance the spontaneity of the patients.

Stretch exercise (1 minute)

Stretching and breathing exercises are used in warm-up calisthenics widely practiced and broadcast on Japanese radio. Exercise often helps patients shake off any drowsiness due to having just eaten, from lacking sufficient sleep, or due to side-effects from medicine.

Self-introduction (2 minutes)

Self-introduction is necessary when the group has a new member. The therapist introduces him- or herself first and the rest of the group follows. To save time, the therapist's self-introduction should be brief, since it will likely be used as the model for the other members of the group.

A short review of the previous art activity (2 minutes)

The therapist asks the members what kind of art activity they did in the previous session. The short review emphasizes the continuity of sessions and enhances the members' motivation in therapy.

Instructions (5–10 minutes)

How the therapist instructs the patients should vary with the patients' function level. In the case of a low-functioning group, dividing the whole process into several small steps and conducting an easy and playful task for a warm-up can reduce patient anxiety.

Making art (20–25 minutes)

It is helpful to conduct deep-breathing and stretching exercises before making art, to calm down restless patients who may have short attention spans. The use of background music while the group is making their art is beneficial because the music can not only relax the patients, but also provide a structure for the therapeutic milieu, and a guide to stay within the time allotted.

Discussion (30 minutes)

One method of conducting the discussion has the therapist seating the group in a circle and letting them put their artwork in the center for everyone to see, and for everyone to be able to easily present their work to the group. If the group members all hesitate to be the first presenter, the therapist may facilitate this process by asking the group, "Which artwork interests you?" During the presentation, the therapist gets the group to describe their feelings about the work and ask questions about other members' artwork.

Feedback (15 minutes)

The therapist instructs the members to review the session and talk freely in the group. The therapist may ask them if they can find similarities and/ or differences between their works of art. This question often facilitates the artwork group review. In this model, the "Discussion" and "Feedback" sections together take up half of the total time available. The running time of these sections should be shortened for low-functioning patients because of their limited attention span.

Closure (5 minutes)

The therapist summarizes the members' comments during feedback. The therapist may address his or her own opinions at the end of sessions. Questionnaires about the art activities and about the therapist's performance as a group facilitator are distributed to the group at the end of each session.

Multi-axial art therapy goals

By keeping in mind the various foci in art therapy, therapists can devise their own themes and art activities. Ault (as cited in Kiempner, 1986), an American art therapist, maintains that the practice of art therapy includes three elements. In this concept, each element has a different therapeutic focus. The first element represents the person-centered approach, which focuses on interpretation of symbols and emotions within an image. The second element represents the process-oriented approach, which focuses on the way the client deals with art materials. The third element represents the product-centered approach, which focuses on increasing the client's ability to control their environment and level of social participation.

In a previous paper (Sezaki, 2007), I expanded on Ault's theory by adding one more axis or focus, "art therapy for assessing patients." In that paper, I detailed the four axes of art therapy goals and how my theory improves upon Ault's. Art activities used for psychological evaluations gained high credibility in Japan; therefore treatment goals based on this focus may be very persuasive for professionals in other fields. The multi-axial treatment theory enables therapists to see the various therapeutic benefits of art and provide creative interventions for their patients. As can be seen in Table 16.1, each axis displays a different focus in art therapy. The therapist can detail the goals of group art therapy and evaluate them periodically within this framework.

A general framework for providing cross-cultural art activities to psychiatric patients can be created from the two concepts briefly described above: theme-oriented and structured approach, and multi-axial goal framework. Application of these two concepts can be seen in the two following case studies. These case studies were conducted in a Japanese psychiatric hospital where I worked as a full-time art therapist. The hospital, which had several occupational therapists and a part-time music therapist, had no art therapy program until I designed it to function as one part of the treatment and rehabilitation plan.

Table 16.1 *Multi-axial goal framework for group art therapy (Sezaki, 2007)*

Axis I Assessment and information (To get client's information and provide a psychological assessment)	Axis II Image expression and communication (To use the image of art as a tool for expressing the self and communicating with others)
Axis III Process of art making (The process of making art has therapeutic benefits)	Axis IV Social activity and recreation (Art activity as a recreation and a lifelong hobby. Creating an artwork to become more socialized)

Case example: Psychiatric inpatient group

Weekly 90-minute art therapy sessions were provided for inpatients in the meeting room of the psychiatric open ward. The room was equipped with a double door and was very quiet. Group members were inpatients who obtained permission from their primary doctors to participate in the therapy. Most of the patients' hospitalizations were short (less than three months). Their diseases and problems varied; some of their diagnoses included schizophrenia, depression, and eating disorders. Each session had an average of 8–10 participants, and occasionally the number exceeded 15. For the group in this case study, the therapist provided two kinds of art activities, theme-oriented and free-choice. During the free-choice activities, group members could choose one of several artistic techniques to express their feelings and thoughts, including free drawing or painting, scribble drawing, clay sculpture, and collage. During the theme-oriented activities, I brought various pieces of art to the group, based upon both client function level and on the therapeutic goals of the session. The multi-axial art therapy goals for this inpatient group were designed as follows.

AXIS I: ASSESSMENT AND INFORMATION

- Assess patient strengths and treatment needs.

- Detect relapses, impulsive behaviors, and suicide ideation in the process of making artwork, and in the final product.

AXIS II: IMAGE EXPRESSION AND COMMUNICATION

- Help patients share their feelings and thoughts regarding hospitalization with others.

- Reduce patients' feelings of loneliness in and out of the hospital.

- Lead patients into the treatment procedures by providing them with a sense of safety and teaching them that therapy is helpful for their recovery.

- Offer the opportunity to help other patients through their own sessions.

- Alleviate patient anxiety by making it easier to express their day-to-day worries.

AXIS III: PROCESS OF ART MAKING

- Promote the healing process through art making and expression.

- Provide an outlet for negative feelings, anger, and irritation in a safe place.

Axis IV: Social activity and recreation

- Help patients gain an interest in continuing their creative activities after being discharged.

Process

In one of the sessions for this group, I provided a therapeutic artwork called "The Monks of Emotion." I thought that the group might enjoy creating a *Teruteru Bozu*, or Sunshine Monk doll, because sculpture had been rarely used during the sessions. A *Teruteru Bozu* is a Japanese folk craft made of white cloth stuffed with cotton and tied off with string to form a head. The benefit of bringing the traditional folk craft to the session revolves around its familiarity and rich implications. This doll is well known as a sort of amulet for bringing fine weather among Japanese people; therefore it can have a metaphorically therapeutic meaning for patients. However, one potentially negative point of this activity is that the doll, which hangs from windows by a thread, could bring to mind thoughts of suicide by hanging. The therapist decided to place the doll on a sink-plunger base instead, and used the activity to have the patients express four emotions: joy, anger, sadness, and pleasure. In Japan, these four are considered to cover the range of human feeling.

Fifteen patients attended the session, including two new members. After conducting a few group activities, including an orientation, the therapist explained the theme of the new activity, and the group members were instructed to choose one of four emotions to create their artwork. Three pieces of large vellum were made into one big sheet of paper with paste. Plastic bags were inflated to a suitable size and used for the monk's head. The plungers, with clay inside the plunge, were fixed to the floor with packing tape. The group used watercolor paints and crayons to decorate the dolls and express their chosen emotional theme. The group members chatted with each other while making their dolls, and their laughter filled the room. After they completed their dolls, which can be seen in Figure 16.1, each small group reviewed the process, and discussed their feelings and thoughts about their artwork. The therapist asked all groups to give a title to their art. This task helped the members become more cohesive. The smaller groups were then brought together to discuss their artwork as a part of the entire group. Each small group selected a member to present their artwork, and the rest of the group supplemented his or her presentation. Other groups gave comments and asked questions.

At the end of the session, the therapist had the entire group review the therapeutic process and their artwork, and finally summarized the comments made by the group.

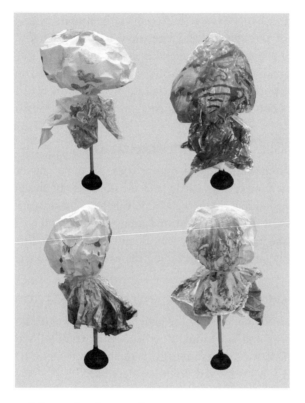

Figure 16.1 *"The Monks of Emotion"*

Discussion

I conducted theme-oriented and structured approach art therapy in this setting for over ten years. The questionnaires completed by the patients suggest that they gained therapeutic benefit from creating their art, and from expressively interacting with other patients. During the "Monks of Emotion" session, one patient commented, "It was the first time I ever laughed so loudly in the hospital." Another patient mentioned, "These exercises gave me the chance to think about the idea of emotion itself." One person, who seemed to develop greater insight into his own emotions, pointed out, "There was a connection among the four feelings...

Joy doesn't exist without sadness. That's why I painted the small image of sadness on the doll of joy." The doll artwork, which allowed the patients to draw facial expressions and paint with watercolors, was an excellent way to facilitate the expression of emotion. Many of the patients commented that they were able to reduce their stress as they expressed their feelings through art, and ultimately felt some relief. The activity also allowed patients to work together and focus on their roles in a small group, and completing the artwork led to a sense of accomplishment. A brief evaluation of the multi-axial art therapy goals for this inpatient group is laid out in the following paragraphs.

Axis I: Assessment and information

Through the artwork created during these sessions, the hospital staff were able to interpret the talents and artistic sense of the patients, and identify some internal conflicts and ambivalences. The artwork sometimes revealed patient suicide ideation, and sometimes even intense hostility on the part of the patient towards their doctor. This provided the staff with clues for early intervention, including the use of seclusion and restraints.

Axis II: Image expression and communication

Artwork was often praised by the patients' peers. Patients also responded to the worries and sufferings of others with words of sympathy and encouragement. In the questionnaire, patients commented: "It was fun," "I got motivated to work," and "I felt less depressed."

Axis III: Process of art making

Many group members commented that making art reduced their stress. Painting and drawing were especially effective. Some comments include "The load on my mind has lightened a little," and "I wish I could do artwork more often."

Axis IV: Social activity and recreation

As yet, there is no information on whether inpatients continued to make art as a hobby. However, many inpatients were happy to continue participating in art therapy day programs after being discharged.

Case example: Alcoholic outpatient group

Bi-weekly 90-minute art therapy sessions were provided for alcoholic patients as a part of their day-care programs. The members chose either art therapy or verbal group meetings, and an average number of 8–10 people participated. The group sessions were sometimes interrupted by telephone calls and visits with other staff because they were held in the hall where outpatients took their lunch. The goals of the alcoholic patient day program included: (a) abstention from drinking; (b) life skill training; (c) explaining communication skills without drinking; (d) developing social skills without drinking; (e) attending regular self-help groups and relating to fellow outpatients; (f) building relationships with support groups and organizations within the community; (g) combating the stigma of alcoholism and hospitalization; and (h) providing cost-efficient treatment to patients (Enomoto, 2005).

With these goals in mind, the author designed the multi-axial art therapy goals for this group of patients as follows.

AXIS I: ASSESSMENT AND INFORMATION

- Assess the patients' strengths and potential and use those strengths to improve their self-esteem and rebuild their pride.

- Detect relapses, impulsive behaviors, and other warning signals in the process of art making and in their final artwork.

AXIS II: IMAGE EXPRESSION AND COMMUNICATION

- Cope with the patients' feelings of loneliness by expressing themselves and sharing with others.

- Rediscover the joy of relating with others through the joint art activities.

- Learn to give and take with others through art making and discussion.

- Help the patients recognize their roles within a group and facilitate appropriate behaviors.

- Develop insight into their drinking habits and other possible problems in their interpersonal relationships.

Axis III: Process of art making

- Reduce the patients' stresses through the process of art making and expression.

- Build adaptability and flexibility through the use of new art materials.

Axis IV: Social activity and recreation

- Help the patients socialize and cultivate good daily habits.

- Help the patients discover hobbies or other activities as a substitute for drinking.

Process

The author devised a therapeutic technique called "The Two Thinkers." Patients were encouraged to draw details of two human-like figures on a large piece of paper. Each figure had a space in which the patients could draw what they thought the figure was thinking, but the piece of paper was folded such that the space could be hidden. On one template, the figures faced each other, and on the other, the figures were back to back. The figures had no hair, eyes, mouths, or clothing. In addition to drawing details of the empty figures, the patients also were given the chance to fill out a personal profile on each figure, including their name, age, occupation, and personal character.

A total of 14 patients came to the session. Sessions usually consisted of both men and women, but this case deals with a session attended by men only. Group members varied in age; some were in their 20s and others were in their 60s, and no attendee had any difficulty in understanding how to create their artwork. Four members chose the face-to-face template, and the rest chose the back-to-back template. After the drawings were completed, the patients presented their artwork to the group individually, and discussed their feelings and thoughts regarding their artwork. The participants who created the pieces shown in Figures 16.2 and 16.3 explained that one of the figures in the picture was himself. The first (Figure 16.2) illustrated a part of his feelings and thoughts regarding his relationship with his female partner. The second (Figure 16.3) illustrated his relationship with a good friend with whom he enjoyed fishing. Nine members of the group drew images representing male–female heterosexual relationships in their artwork. One participant described the figures as a child and a parent. The artwork helped the participants learn more about each other in a warm atmosphere.

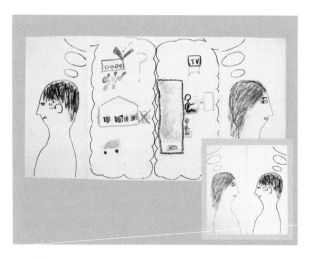

Figure 16.2 *"The Two Thinkers" (1)*

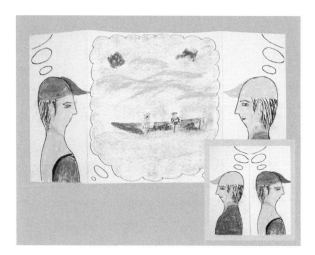

Figure 16.3 *"The Two Thinkers" (2)*

Discussion

The practice of conducting art therapy in this group setting has been ongoing for eight years. Many techniques and materials have been utilized for the theme-oriented art activities, including puppet making, mono-prints, and drawing games. The members in this group maintain high physical and cognitive function, which made them able to explore their insights into their problems and strengths while enjoying a variety of creative activities. In the artwork "The Two Thinkers," the members expressed their feelings and thoughts regarding interpersonal relationships through drawing. This playful technique seemed to facilitate self-disclosure on the part of the patients. Six of the 14 participants stated that one of the figures in the picture was themselves, and others also implied they expressed a part of themselves through their art. The therapist noticed that many patients using the back-to-back template portrayed the figures as thinking the same thing. The therapist made the assumption that those images showed the participants' desire to be close to others. There is a possibility that the back-to-back template was considered to be easier to complete because it required only one space to be filled.

The theme of this activity evoked a number of responses from group members. Their imagination and senses of humor warmed up the whole group. The therapist posed a number of questions to the group, including "If you could say something to the two figures in the picture, what would it be?," to help the participants gain insight into their interpersonal relationships. A brief evaluation of the multi-axial art therapy goals for this patient group is laid out in the following paragraphs.

AXIS I: ASSESSMENT AND INFORMATION

A lower level of detail and poor content in artwork often indicated that the patient continued to have a hidden drinking habit. The artwork of those patients was also useful in assessing function and in detecting the early stages of depression.

AXIS II: IMAGE EXPRESSION AND COMMUNICATION

Participants who had kept themselves from drinking, and had rebuilt their relationships with others, created richer images, and described them more fluently and articulately. The therapist recognized that some artistic activities, such as joint paintings, were especially helpful in developing participants' sense of give-and-take, and also helped the participants examine their own roles within a group setting.

AXIS III: PROCESS OF ART MAKING

Patient comments and behavior both confirmed that the action of expressing themselves through art was helpful in reducing their stress and alleviating their suffering.

AXIS IV: SOCIAL ACTIVITY AND RECREATION

Some participants enjoyed ceramics class and their creations were sold at various events. For recreation, the members also enjoyed making a calendar in which images representing each month were created in collage.

Conclusion

Sprayregen (1989) contends, "Art therapists are most able to meet the challenges of conducting brief art therapy groups when prepared with clearly conceptualized group rationales, structures, and objectives" (p.17). She also emphasized periodic review of group goals, and willingness to commit necessary revisions, in order to work with psychiatric patients in groups. These remarks are relevant to the issue of providing cross-cultural art activities to Japanese psychiatric patients. Although the two concepts mentioned in this chapter—theme-oriented and structured approach, and multi-axial goal framework—have not been fully researched, they have been shown over a long period to be effective with Japanese patients.

On some levels, cultural and ethnic differences can affect the process and outcome of psychotherapies with patients who have non-Western backgrounds. However, creativity transcends borders, and can help therapists to analyze better patient needs and to provide more effective interventions. It is our conviction that we can serve people of all ages, races, and ethnic backgrounds through art, which possesses a universality recognized by people worldwide.

Acknowledgements

A very special acknowledgement is due to Dr. Yutaka Akimoto, the chairman of the board of trustees, Rikou-kai medical cooperation, whose generosity and encouragement are deeply appreciated.

References

Case, C. and Dalley, T. (1992) *The Handbook of Art Therapy*. London: Routledge.

Enomoto, M. (2005) *Enomoto Minoru Chosaku Shu 3* [Enomoto Minoru Writing Collection 3]. Tokyo, Japan: Nihon Hyoron Sha.

Iwai, H., Horii, A. and Ito, N. (1985) "Gurûpu âto serapî: byouga setumei yakuwari koukan hou" [Group art therapy: Picture explaining and role exchange technique]. *Geijyutu Ryouhou: Nihon Geijyutu Ryouhou Gakkai Shi 16*, 33–39.

Kiempner, Y. (Producer/Director) (1986) *Art Therapy: The Healing Vision with R. Ault and Y. Kiempner* [Video Recording]. Topeka, KS: The Menninger Foundation.

Liebmann, M. (1986) *Art Therapy for Groups: A Handbook of Themes, Games and Exercises*. Cambridge, MA: Brookline Books.

Mine, Y., Kato, K., Ito, Y., Nomura, T., Takahashi, T. and Aizawa, S. (1991) "Shûdan kaiga ryoho ni okeru utu jyoutai kanjya no kaigahyougen no oudanteki tokuchou" [Characteristic drawings and clinical stages in cases of depressive patients]. *Geijyutu Ryouhou: Nihon Geijyutu Ryouhou Gakkai Shi 22*, 1, 31–41.

Reynolds, D.K. (1989) *Flowing Bridges, Quiet Waters: Japanese Psychotherapies, Morita and Naikan*. Albany, NY: State University of New York Press.

Sezaki, S. (2007) *Souzouteki Âto Serapî* [Creative Art Therapy]. Nagoya, Japan: Reimei Shobo.

Sezaki, S. and Bloomgarden, J. (2000) "Home-based art therapy for older adults." *Art Therapy: Journal of the American Art Therapy Association 17*, 4, 283–290.

Sprayregan, B. (1989) "Brief inpatient group: A conceptual design for art therapist." *American Journal of Art Therapy 28*, 1, 13–17.

Sue, D.W. and Sue, D. (1990) *Counseling the Culturally Different: Theory and Practice*, 2nd edn. New York, NY: John Wiley.

Walsh, R. (1989) "Asian Psychotherapies." In: R.J. Corsini and D. Wedding (eds) *Current Psychotherapies*, 4th edn (pp.547–559). Itasca, IL: F.E. Peacock.

Yalom, I. (1983) *Inpatient Group Psychotherapy*. New York, NY: Basic Books.

Chapter 17

Affective Color Symbolism and Markers Cosplay

Standardized Procedure for Clinical Assessment

Liona Lu

Issues of "should or should not" or "how" to interpret a client's artworks have long been of interest for many art therapists (Allen, 1995, 2005; Gantt, 1992; Moon, 2002). Colors in pictures, too, have drawn the attention of scholars and therapists. Rorschach (1942; Schachtel, 1943) regarded it a psychodiagnostic method and assumed that there was a systematic relationship between the perception of color and emotional response. Following this trend, there are many studies concerning color as a diagnostic element (Allison, Blatt and Zimet, 1968; Kim *et al.*, 2011; Shapiro, 1977; Siipola, 1950). In the field of art therapy, attempting to understand the complexity and richness of the visual sensation of color remains a great concern (Levy, 1980; Riley, 1995).

Stressing the importance of understanding color in recent years, there have been several studies concerning computerized systems to evaluate colors in drawings for psychological assessment (Kim, 2008b; Kim, Bae and Lee, 2007). Schafer (1949) stressed that psychological thinking can never be replaced by a scoring system and an ideal objective assessment should be accompanied by clinical insight; while Lichtenberger (2006) considered just comparing numbers to base rates to be insufficient in assessment. Many art-based instruments of this kind may be incapable of measuring many of the variables humans present, so clinicians should recognize that the scoring-based instruments are supplemental tools for analyzing, processing, and storing vast amounts of data quickly and efficiently (Reynolds, 2000). Subjective but trained clinical judgment is more appropriate for processing the comprehensive nature of clients (Mattson, 2010). Jung (1960) believed that images speak for themselves and there is no need for interpretation. Furthermore, it may never be possible to determine what colors signify. With the long debate of whether or not images can be read or rated, there is an increasing consensus that a combination of both subjective and objective methods for art-based assessment could benefit the field of art therapy (Kapitan, 2007; Kim, 2008a; Mattson, 2009, 2010).

Collecting a client's Affective Color Symbolism (ACS) information during the first interview or in the beginning sessions is a technique that the author developed during the 1990s. Inspired by how pre-school-age children use colors in their drawings (Lowenfeld and Brittain, 1987), ACS was based on the findings concerning children's color concept, and the author's clinical practice for the past 22 years (Lu, 2011).

Color preferences indicate emotional reactions (Zentner, 2001) in that they elicit positive or negative feelings (Kaya and Epps, 2004). As an example, children tend to use their more preferred colors for the nice figures and their less preferred colors for the nasty figures (Burkitt, Barrett and Davis, 2003). The affective tendency of color depends directly upon the intensity of its pleasantness or unpleasantness (Yokoyama, 1921). ACS is designed to obtain a client's most preferred and least preferred colors in a hierarchical manner and to get some affect-elicit colors chosen through symbolic association.

With a person-centered, phenomenological, and dynamic-oriented therapy approach in developing these assessment tools, the author does not intend to state that there is a specific relationship between a color and a corresponding emotion. On the contrary, the client's color choice is respected and considered as valuable information. Interpretation should only be addressed along with other presented information in the assessment session, verbal and non-verbal, including the client's personal history. Although some colors seem highly preferred by everyone (Adams and Osgood, 1973), there is conflicting evidence whether color preference is related to culture (Saito, 1996). This chapter will focus on the procedures of ACS and its derivation, Markers Cosplay (MC), with an aim to improve the therapy quality by enhancing the therapist empathetic ability as well as the client's insight.

Affective color symbolism and markers cosplay

ACS and MC were developed as a pair of assessment tools to be used in an interview or other sessions with those who have achieved the "preschematic stage," when simple shapes such as encephalopods and others start appearing in their drawings (more than four years old).

Administration concerns and procedures

In ACS, the client is provided with a box of color markers and invited to choose the three most preferred and the three least preferred markers and arranged in a hierarchical manner. To elicit the client's self-concept and other value-related information, the client also identifies the most powerful marker, the most vulnerable marker, and any other affect-elicit marker that may be of interest for that specific client. After each choice, the client returns the chosen marker to the box, so that there are always 12 colors to choose from each time. This step is intended to allow clients to choose the color more than once to represent other conditions or individuals. To make it more fun, use terms like "good guys" and "bad guys" instead of the most preferred and the least preferred when working with school-age children. The client is encouraged to answer the questions of how a particular marker is powerful or vulnerable when the choice is made.

In MC, the markers are used as toys with the colors serving to create characters in a scene. This procedure encourages spontaneous play. MC can be applied before or after the client's ACS data are collected in the same session, but only with a certain interval in between. In an interview session, MC is centered on the family situation. The client chooses a colored paper from a package of 12 colors to represent the family's space. Then from the box of color markers, the client chooses one marker to represent each family member, *one by one*. The therapist uses the chosen markers to color the client's family genogram and takes digital photos of the final family scene.

Materials

In collecting a client's ACS, a box of 12, 16, or 18 colored markers or any brand of any minimum size of drawing materials that includes the following nine colors is used: red, orange, yellow, yellow-green or light green, green, green-blue or light blue, blue, purple, brown, and the three achromatic colors—white, gray, and black. Ideally, the markers or drawing materials should each have an identical appearance, be large, easy to hold, and not produce any mess. In MC, a package of colored papers (39 × 27 cm) with the 12 mentioned colors for selection to represent the client's "specific" space is required.

Rationale

The use of color in ACS and MC is based on the assumption that "individuals more or less unconsciously attribute their own characteristics, feelings and motives to non-human and inanimate objects" (Ogden, 2001, p.107). From a psychodynamic perspective, the inner states are externalized or projected into arts media and transformation becomes possible (Johnson, 1998). Even though color is closely related to emotions and feelings, caution needs to be paid when interpreting a client's use of color. Color meaning in ACS and MC should be understood using the client's stated associations.

In ACS, color is regarded as a medium for expression rather than a diagnostic tool. In keeping with this notion, color preferences are considered a primary process, in which the mental processes are directly related to the functions of the id. Considerable empirical studies demonstrate the impact of color on our emotions (Boyatzis and Varghese, 1994; Cimbalo, Beck and Sendziak, 1978; Hemphill, 1996; Linton, 1999; Saito, 1996; Valdez and Mehrabian, 1994; Wexner, 1982). The emotional use of color in expressionism is an example of the primary process.

"Stationary color" is defined as the color of the object perceived in normal conditions (Lowenfeld and Brittain, 1987). Young children tend to use colors according to their emotional needs before their Stationary Color Concept (SCC) is greatly developed, and gradually and consistently applied in their drawings around age seven. A study in Taiwan involving approximately 1600 four to nine-year-old children's drawings indicated that children's SCC grows gradually with time and that Lowenfeld's theory with respect to color development for four to nine-year-old children is applicable in a Taiwanese context (Lu, 1998a, 1998b, 2005/2009). The use of SCC is an example of a "secondary process" in which the mental process is directly related to the functions of the ego.

The author assumes that color use in drawings reflects the process and the struggle between one's subjective (primary process or id) and objective (secondary process or ego) parts of mentality (Lu, 2005/2009). When SCC is applied to a particular item of a drawing, it signifies the recognition of that item in reality. Thus, the artist's consistent use of a stationary color suggests a fairly good sense of reality testing. While the subjective use of color in younger children is natural, when it occurs in drawings by older children, it may suggest symbolic or sentimental meaning. In ACS and MC, one's color choice is governed according to the symbolic link to the internalized roles. However, SCC may still be used, especially for Schematic Stage children. Given that children had already completed their ACS, if they choose to adhere to their SCC during MC, it may indicate a psychological distancing or reluctance to express themselves.

Special consideration in administering ACS and MC

It is hoped that people who use this projective technique have a thorough grounding in color psychology and clinical psychology which includes personality theory, developmental psychology, abnormal psychology, an understanding of the dynamics of adjusting, and family theories. School teachers are encouraged to use it after proper trainings.

Although not unusual, a client's indecisiveness or change of color for a specific member in MC or any spontaneous response initiated during the process should be noted and is a valuable part of the client's total response. The actualization of ACS and MC creates a psychological space—a hybrid of one's past, present, and future, real and imaginary—in which one travels at one's own pace. A shift of choice implies a change of perceived relationship or emotional atmosphere with that particular person.

Maximum benefits occur during the first use of this technique. It can be applied in any session, or just for an assessment combined with other psychological measures. Whether ACS or family MC should be administered first depends mostly upon the therapist's school, experience, and personal style. The sequence may or may not make any difference if only the client's resistance or defense is considered.

Clinical use and discussion of ACS and MC

ACS and MC can be used during discharge or as pre- and post-evaluation tools. The client's consistency of ACS across time suggests the credibility of this tool (Chang, 2011). From the author's experience, the client's most and least preferred colors seldom change except in hierarchical order. If a large change occurs, it may suggest malingering or a total personality change. However, the most powerful and the most vulnerable colors, and colors that represent family members, may change as long as one's affect or attitude toward that person or life philosophy is modified. It is not unusual that this change may happen in a single-day workshop in which ACS and MC is collected as a pre- and post-evaluation tool.

After group trust has been developed, ACS can be administered in a group form, although it was originally designed for single-subject administration. MC can be modified to a drawing task, in which each member is represented by one colored geometric shape. This single activity or its pre- and post-versions often invite group discussion. Using ACS and MC regularly for psychological evaluation makes it possible to compile a library of data. When very specific thematic material must be elicited, MC can be centered in the particular place; thus classroom MC, office MC, dorm MC, and so on take place.

Making a colored genogram instead of the traditional one using the client's ACS helps the therapist recognize or review the client's process. In clinical settings or case conferences, the use of colored genograms with ACS data generates consensus among multidisciplinary staff. Clients' artworks can be understood empathetically, so that art therapy communicates to other clinical colleagues and administrators.

As it is difficult to conceive life without a multitude of colors in nature and daily life, ACS and MC heighten clients' self-awareness by relating different aspects of the self to colors. This use of color as a language for self-expression and reflection may also inform daily life and art appreciation. It may be in this fashion that color is regarded as one of the most important components of our internal existence (Vendler, 1995 as cited in Clark, 2004).

Case example: Laurie

Laurie (pseudonym), aged eight years and three months, and moderately hearing impaired, was brought to art therapy for her short attention span, poor concentration in class, and extreme obsession with the popular Japanese manga characters, the Pearl Mermaids. The first and the only time the therapist saw her, she was apparently angry with her mother for bringing her to a strange place. The pair of glasses she wore that magnified her expressive and shining eyes suggested a sight problem. Laurie is the second child of the family, and was born and raised abroad when her father attended a professional training program in North America. There were complications during her birth, but her hearing impairment was not found till aged three. The family returned to Taiwan the same year and had lived with the paternal grandmother since she was three years old. A maid attended to the grandmother. Laurie had a talented 18-year-old sister who had "no time for her" because of heavy school work. Although her parents were busy in their respective careers, they were concerned about Laurie's condition and brought her to therapy on a weekday afternoon.

Believing that the parents may gain insight from observing how their child behaved or interacted with the therapist and after careful consideration of the parents' background, Laurie's parents were invited to observe on the monitor in the observation room. The interview session with Laurie took an hour and a half, and the after-session discussion with the parents took half an hour. Laurie was left to draw whatever she liked while the therapist joined the parents in the observation room.

Although Laurie entered the therapy room shouting angrily, she was quite cooperative in the session. When asked how she went home and what she usually did after school, she replied that she walked home by herself and always found herself "alone." (The parents reported that the school was across the road and a brief walk away, and the grandmother and maid were at home, or in the garden.) She also complained that her parents did not allow her to watch *Pearl Mermaids* on TV, and, worse, her freedom to access that program on the web was restricted, too.

Laurie's ACS information

After a brief conversation, she was asked to choose from a box of 12 colored markers: the three most preferred, the three least preferred, the most powerful, and the most vulnerable. Laurie's three preferred colors were pink (herself, later), light blue (sister, later), and purple; the least preferred, black, brown, and dark green. She chose dark blue as the most powerful color and orange for the most vulnerable, which was the color chosen for the maid later. Laurie spontaneously asked to choose the cool color. When asked "The coolest color?" she replied, "No, just cool." She chose light green for that, which was the color for her mother later. To have a better understanding of Laurie's ACS representation, her family genogram is colored according to her later MC and presented together in Figure 17.1.

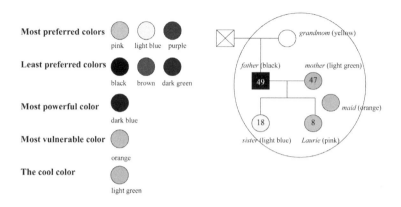

Figure 17.1 *Laurie's ACS data and color family genogram*

Laurie's drawings

Following the ACS, she was directed to make a Human Figure Drawing (HFD) (Figure 17.2) and a Free Drawing (FD) on A4-size papers. Laurie's HFD depicts a long-haired girl, with appearance and clothing obviously resembling characters in *Pearl Mermaids*. The line quality, the geometric shapes, and well-proportioned figure indicate age-appropriate functioning. The overlapping tendency of shapes, a characteristic of the Schematic Stage, is shown in many aspects of this drawing, such as the overall hair against the body, the bunch of front hair against the left arm, and the layers of hair. Though not completely successful or logical in solving the spatial problem, Laurie's HFD indicates an eight to nine-year-old intellectual functioning. The deliberately treated hair and pieces of clothing and the stressed collarbones may imply her fascination with this subject, and the wide stance of the figure may suggest "an aggressive defiance of authority and/or insecurity being defended, sometimes by acting out" (Ogden, 2001, p.92).

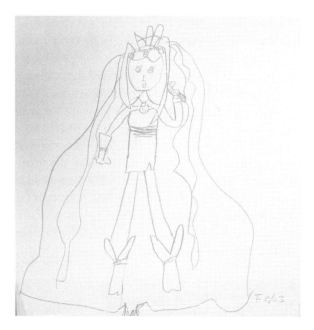

Figure 17.2 *Laurie's Human Figure Drawing*

In post-interrogations about her HFD, Laurie stated that the 15-year-old Mermaid Princess Ai-Li was looking for her lost pearl in the human world. She liked singing, eating bubbles, and making crowns out of flowers; she had many good human friends. As singing is the most powerful weapon for the mermaids, Ai-Li was depicted armed and singing "beautifully" against the enemy. Laurie's FD depicted another princess of *Pearl Mermaids* in a farm scene.

The rather impulsive line quality may be a result of the length of time that had passed, rather than an indication of pathology, because otherwise this picture is carefully delineated and colored. Again, the SCC and stereotyped subject matter applied in this drawing suggest normal Schematic Stage functioning. Laurie drew with enthusiasm, actively revealing the princess's story.

Laurie's MC

Lastly, she was encouraged to play out a family scene using the colored markers and objects available on the table (Figure 17.3). Laurie chose pink to represent her family space. She added a transparent brown plastic board on the right side as the family's living room. Her choice of colors for family members were played out in a dramatic scenario—*I (pink) am coming home...* (moving the marker from the living room to her room); *the maid (orange) is accompanying grandma (yellow) watching TV*; *Sis is coming home very late...* (moving the light blue marker toward the left side and placed in the same line with the pink marker, but with her head in the opposite direction); *Mother (light green) is coming home* (moving the marker toward the left side and placing it closely parallel to the sister and opposite to the one that represents herself; *the merciless Father* (an exaggerated tone) *is coming home exhausted...he joins the grandma watching TV.* (First she chose *black* but later played with *gray*.) The family is obviously divided into two groups (Figure 17.3). On the left side she had pink (self), light green (mother), and light blue (sister) markers. On the right side, she placed the orange (maid), yellow (grandmother), and gray (father) markers in a top to bottom, left to right order respectively.

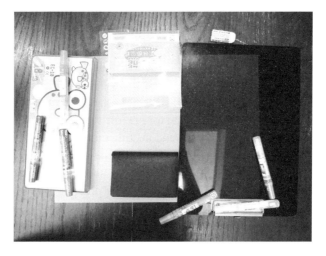

Figure 17.3 *Laurie's marker cosplay*

Post-session discussion with parents

Mother acknowledged that Laurie used mother's favorite color, green, to represent the mother and felt sorry for being seen as cool by her daughter; Laurie's singing defect was compensated as Princess Ai-Li could sing delightfully. Mother mentioned her job situation and was thinking about quitting her job in order to have more time with Laurie. The maid used to throw away the full floor of mermaid drawings Laurie produced when cleaning her room. The more limits set, the more emotional needs or obsessions grew. Both parents gained lots of insight from the observation process. When all returned to join Laurie in the therapy room, she procrastinated about going home, although two hours had already passed. Laurie refused to leave the original HFD and FD for the author's therapy record. Instead, she left the other two mermaid drawings that she drew when the therapist was away.

Interpretation

From Laurie's HFD and FD, age-appropriate functioning is suggested. Although it is not unusual that Schematic Stage children draw the stereotyped subject, her extreme obsession with *Pearl Mermaids* may be reinforced by her loneliness and the parents' restrictions against that fantasy world, which may be responsible for her attention deficit and impulsivity. Her identification with the mermaid princess compensates for her incapability to sing well and lack of good friends in reality. It may be in the therapy room at that specific moment that her fantasy was recognized and contained, and her anger and complaints were released through the expressive family MC. Laurie's spontaneous adding of the "cool" color, her mother's favorite color and a choice from the secondary process, suggests the importance of her mother to her and a conflicted feeling toward her. On the contrary, the colors for her father are subjective (primary process), and the change of color from black to gray indicates an insight generated through MC while she was allowed to examine her relationship with each family member more objectively. As one's self-concept is shaped gradually from how one has been treated by significant others, the use of Laurie's most favored color for herself and for her family space indicated a positive self-concept and perceived warm family atmosphere. Further, the parents' insight and reaction meant there was no need for more therapy.

Conclusion

ACS and MC can be applied to any population by a wide variety of mental health professionals and is useful to clinicians in a variety of ways. The brief and clear instruction of ACS and MC allow the client to express his or her positive and negative feelings with ease while the collected data enable an objective understanding of later artworks. Those whose "intuition" plays an important role in art therapy will find ACS and MC great aids in understanding the client and their art in depth. In MC, the reflective space created through color selection provides opportunities to reevaluate, reassure, or reinforce the faith one has about certain relationships. It is expected that both therapist and client gain insight through this interactive and playful procedure.

Even though art therapy embraces a wide spectrum of approaches from the art as therapy to art psychotherapy, all believe in the healing power of art. If art reveals itself to the artist, ACS and MC help channel some of the unconscious material into a conscious level, allowing it to be heard. When working with children, it is one of the very few effective assessment tools which can be used in less-developed regions or crisis situations as the space and equipment needed is minimal and adaptable to different settings.

References

Adams, F.M. and Osgood, C.E. (1973) "A cross-cultural study of three colors in an office interior on mood and performance." *Perceptual and Motor Skills 76*, 235–241.

Allen, P. (1995) *Art is a Way of Knowing.* Boston, MA: Shambhala.

Allen, P. (2005) *Art is a Spiritual Path: Engaging the Sacred through the Practice of Art and Writing.* Boston: Shambhala.

Allison, J., Blatt, S.J. and Zimet, C.N. (1968) *The Interpretation of Psychological Tests.* New York, NY: Harper and Row.

Boyatzis, C.J. and Varghese, R. (1994) "Children's emotional associations with colors." *Journal of Genetic Psychology 155*, 1, 77–87.

Burkitt, E., Barrett, M. and Davis, A. (2003) "Children's color choices for completing drawings of affectively characterized topics." *Journal of Child Psychology and Psychiatry 44*, 3, 445–455.

Chang, Y.M. (2011) *The Project Development and Effectiveness of Filial Art Therapy Group.* Unpublished master's paper. Graduate Art Therapy Program, Taipei University of Education [written in Chinese].

Cimbalo, R.S., Beck, K.L. and Sendziak, D.S. (1978) "Emotionally toned pictures and color selection for children and college students." *Journal of Genetic Psychology 133*, 303–304.

Clark, A.J. (2004) "On the meaning of color in early recollections." *Journal of Individual Psychology 60*, 2, 141–155.

Gantt, L. (1992) "A Description and History of Art Therapy Assessment in Research." In: H. Wadeson (ed.) *A Guide to Conducting Art Therapy Research* (pp.120–140). Mundelein, IL: The American Art Therapy Association.

Hemphill, M. (1996) "A note on adults' color–emotion associations." *Journal of Genetic Psychology 157*, 275–181.

Johnson, D.R. (1998) "On the therapeutic action of the creative arts therapies: The psychodynamic model." *The Arts in Psychotherapy 25*, 2, 85–99.

Jung, C. (1960) *The Transcendent Function.* Princeton, NJ: Bollingen.

Kapitan, L. (2007) "Will art therapy cross the digital culture divide?" *Art Therapy: Journal of the American Art Therapy Association 24*, 2, 50–51.

Kaya, N. and Epps, H.H. (2004) "Relationship between color and emotion: A study of college students." *College Student Journal 38*, 3, 396–405.

Kim, S.I. (2008a) "Art therapy [letter to the editor]." *Art Therapy: Journal of the American Art Therapy Association 25*, 1, 41.

Kim, S.I. (2008b) "Computer judgment of main color in a drawing for art psychotherapy assessment." *The Arts in Psychotherapy 35*, 2, 140–150.

Kim, S.I., Bae, J. and Lee, Y. (2007) "A computer system to rate the color-related formal elements in art therapy assessment." *The Arts in Psychotherapy 34*, 3, 223–237.

Kim, S.I., Han, J., Kim, Y.H. and Oh, Y.J. (2011) "A Computer Art Therapy System for Kinetic Family Drawing (CATS_KFD)." *The Arts in Psychotherapy 38*, 1, 17–28.

Levy, B.I. (1980) "Research into the psychological meaning of color." *American Journal of Art Therapy 19*, 87–91.

Lichtenberger, E.O. (2006) "Computer utilization and clinical judgment in psychological assessment reports." *Journal of Clinical Psychology 13*, 328–334.

Linton, H. (1999) *Color in Architecture: Design Methods for Buildings, Interiors and Urban Space.* New York, NY: McGraw Hill.

Lowenfeld, V. and Brittain, W.L. (1987) *Creative and Mental Growth*, 8th edn. New York, NY: Macmillan.

Lu, L. (2011) "Affective Color Symbolism (ACS) and Family Markers Cosplay (FMC) as Diagnostic Tools in the First Art Therapy Interview." Paper presented at the Korea Arts Therapy Institute Spring Conference, National Youth Center of Korea, South Korea, 21 May.

Lu, Y.C. (1998a) *Study of the Development of Children's Color Concept through Their Drawings.* Taipei: Chinese Color Research Press [written in Chinese].

Lu, Y.C. (1998b) "The Use of Color in Children's Drawings." 1998 "Color and Life" Conference, proceedings published by National Taiwan Art Education Archive [written in Chinese].

Lu, Y.C. (2005/2009) *Art Therapy: Interpretation of Drawings—Understanding Children through Their Arts*, 3rd edn. Taipei: Psychological Publisher [written in Chinese]/ Sichuan: Chon-chin University Press [written in simplified Chinese].

Mattson, D.C. (2009) "Accessible image analysis for art assessment." *The Arts in Psychotherapy 6*, 4, 208–213.

Mattson, D.C. (2010) "Issues in computerized art therapy assessment." *The Arts in Psychotherapy 37*, 4, 328–334.

Moon, C. (2002) *Studio Art Therapy: Cultivating the Artist Identity in the Art Therapist.* London: Jessica Kingsley Publishers.

Ogden, D.P. (2001) *Psychodiagnostics and Personality Assessment*, 3rd edn. Los Angeles, CA: Western Psychological Services.

Reynolds, C.R. (2000) "The use of computer for making judgments and decisions" [special issue]. *Psychological Assessment 12*, 3–111.

Riley, C.A. (1995) *Color Codes: Modern Theories of Color in Philosophy, Painting, Architecture, Literature, Music and Psychology.* Hanover, NH: University Press of New England.

Rorschach, H. (1942) *Psychodiagnostics: A Diagnostic Test Based on Perception.* New York, NY: Grune and Stratton.

Saito, M. (1996) "Comparative studies on color preference in Japan and other Asian regions, with special emphasis on the preference for white." *Color Research and Application 21*, 1, 35–49.

Schachtel, E.G. (1943) "On color and affect: Contributions to an understanding of Rorschach's Test II." *Psychiatry 6*, 393–409.

Schafer, R. (1949) "Psychological tests in clinical research." *Journal of Consulting Psychology 13*, 328–334.

Shapiro, D. (1977) "A Perceptual Understanding of Color Response, 2nd edn." In: M.A. Rickers-Ovsiankina (ed.) *Rorschach Psychology* (pp.251–301). Huntington, NY: Robert E. Krieger Publishing.

Siipola, E.M. (1950) "The influence of color on reactions to ink blots." *Journal of Personality 18*, 358–382.

Valdez, P. and Mehrabian, A. (1994) "Effects of color on emotions." *Journal of Experimental Psychology: General 123*, 394–409.

Wexner, L.B. (1982) "The degree to which colors are associated with mood-tones." *Journal of Applied Psychology 6*, 432–435.

Yokoyama, M. (1921) "Affective tendency as conditioned by color and form." *American Journal of Psychology 32*, 81–107.

Zentner, M.R. (2001) "Preference for colour and colour–emotion combination in early childhood." *Developmental Science 4*, 4, 389–398.

Chapter 18

Integrating Person-Centered Expressive Arts with Chinese Metaphors

Fiona Chang

Expressive arts therapy, like spices, originated far away from Hong Kong. When we blend expressive arts therapy into a Chinese community practice, it is important to "mix" them into the local context. One needs to consider the Chinese culture—arts, metaphors, values, and beliefs—so that the most appealing taste emerges. In this chapter, I share my experience of blending expressive arts therapy with a person-centered approach and the Chinese culture.

Benefits of using arts in the Chinese community

I grew up with the belief that emotions disturb the balance of our body–mind–spirit connection. The prominent style of relating to emotions in Chinese culture is to preserve social harmony and down-play emotional displays (Mortenson, 1999). To hold these deep-rooted values, we sometimes avoid, reject, and hide our true feelings. Such subtle suppression inhibits the congruence in human interaction and our true being. In Chinese culture there is a tendency to look for socially acceptable ways to manage buried emotions. Since ancient times, painting, music, and poetry have been used as an outlet. Expressive arts are safe alternatives of authentic expression for connecting our inner and outer reality: body, mind, and spirit (Rogers, 1993; Samuels and Lane, 1998). Arts can also enhance communication effectively and authentically (Malchiodi, 2005; McNiff, 1981).

Each individual has a distinctive response to each different art form. It is therefore vital to incorporate a variety of art forms to experience their unique quality. When people are not familiar with the arts, it helps to provide choices for spontaneous experimenting and locating their comfortable modalities. I favor Person-Centered Expressive Arts Therapy (PCEAT) because the integrated use of arts gives a sense of autonomy, allows holistic exploration, and facilitates integration of our body–emotion–mind–spirit (Rogers, 1993). The process of creative connection by mixed creative modalities can be visualized as a spiral, plumbing the depth of our body, mind, emotions, and spirit, which brings us to our wellspring of creative vitality.

Such enhancement of our whole body–mind–emotions–spirit system synchronizes with the holistic concept of the body–mind–spirit connection in Traditional Chinese Medicine. In Confucianism and Taoism, the manifestation of equilibrium or the state of harmony is that "All things are nourished together without their injuring one another" (Cheng, 2000, p.6). Cheng added that a harmonious relationship can be established by congruent communication. Through visualization and sensation by the arts in person-centered communication, we can express feelings in a congruent way. PCEAT emphasizes the importance of deep understanding with empathetic listening, non-judgmental compassion, and mutual respect. It is in line with the Chinese culture of having harmony. We aim at fostering self-actualization of each individual, widening the scope of understanding, finding one's true needs, and transforming the negative energy into healing resources for a positive change. In that process, we never analyze or interpret art. Interpreting the art of a client gives the authority to the interpreter and fosters a dependent relationship on the therapist. It may even demean the ability of clients to understand their own art. Based on these values, we create a respectful climate of understanding so that the artist-clients can find their own meaning.

Use of Chinese metaphors in expressive arts

To utilize the benefits of arts and infuse Chinese culture locally, I select Chinese metaphors as themes of creative exploration in PCEAT. The following examples are from the expressive arts programs I conducted in public hospitals with adults with health challenges.

"Wu Xing" 五行—The Five Elements of Nature

We express our emotions in different ways—articulated in words, expressed through non-verbal language, or "spoken" in silence. As we grow older, we contain our emotions inside us consciously or unconsciously. These suppressed emotions may affect our wellbeing and as such it may benefit us to unfold, filter, and clear them.

In Chinese cosmology, philosophy, and medical theory, the Five Elements of Nature, "Wu Xing," describe the fundamental processes of nature (Rossi, Caretto and Scheid, 2007). They are, conceptually, Water, Wood, Fire, Earth, and Metal. The stability of an element is affected by a specific emotion. In Traditional Chinese Medicine, the imbalance of these elements poses a negative impact on health (Table 18.1).

Table 18.1 *The Five Elements*

Element of "Wu Xing"	Emotion	Affected human organ
Water	Fear	Kidney/Bladder
Wood	Anger	Liver/Gall bladder
Fire	Joy/Indulgence	Heart/Small intestine
Earth	Pensiveness/Worry	Spleen/Stomach
Metal	Sadness	Lung/Large intestine

A balanced "Five Elements" brings harmony and good health (Levitt, 2000). Harmony in our body–mind–thought–spirit could be achieved better by expressing and unfolding the emotions. The creative process begins with stimulation of the senses by exploring representations of the Five Elements. Nature-based materials (wood, sand, stone, tree branches, water, soil, etc.) provide a sensory experience inspired by their qualities (Moon, 2010). As suggested by Rappaport (2009), listening to the body opens the doorway to the body's wisdom and brings the next steps toward growth and healing.

There has been no scientific study on the association of the Five Elements to human emotions. Nevertheless there is a rationale underpinning further investigation. Using these as a metaphor to describe emotions, and stimulate thinking and creating, is a pragmatic way of introducing arts in a Chinese community. Whether each element truly represents any particular emotion does not really matter; this is the trigger to creative expression and exploration. At the end it is for the therapist and the creator to understand the personal meanings of each element and listen to the hidden message in the process. The objectives of the "Wu Xing" workshop were:

1. to be conscious of the Five Elements of our feelings and their connection with the body, mind, and spirit

2. to understand our deeper feelings through the arts

3. to accept and let go the emotions at the pace of the participants.

At the start, the participants were invited to select at least one object that related to each of the Five Elements (Figure 18.1). They could select one with a quality related to their personality and their here-and-now feelings. They felt, touched, smelled, and explored each object. If they did not have any idea, they could just pick up the one that captured their attention or let the elements speak to them. After sharing, they would unfold their emotions through visual art, creative exploration, and dialoguing with the element. My support through accepting eye contact and a caring gesture affirmed the autonomy of each to create, to express, and to release their feelings. The genuine presence of the participants and the therapist served to provide a safe environment for the experimentation within the art-making process. All the physical and psychological responses to the creative exploration were hints for self-understanding.

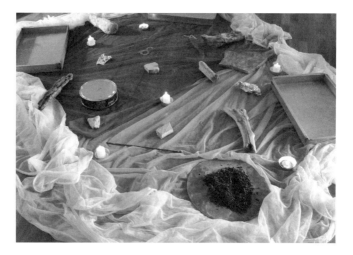

Figure 18.1 *The Five Elements*

The art-making process was then crystallized and consolidated through writing. The participants used both their dominant and non-dominant hands to write about their unfolding creative journey. The closing ritual for the session focused on giving thanks to the elements. Each participant took a turn to say, "Thanks to you [name of the element], I have learnt…" The workshop ended with holding hands to feel the healing energy circulating among us. The participants truly felt the group support. Finally, we imagined using our hands to scoop water from the wellspring and clean ourselves from head to toe. We were refueled by the vitality of this imaginary water. Our body–mind–spirit–soul was totally refreshed. We could feel our new selves.

The exploratory process becomes more powerful when we try mixing visual art with different modalities. In the "Wu Xing" group, the participants added voices, sounds, and movement to their images. They also wrote about the process as a means to dialogue with the images, sounds, and gesture. The writing process seemed to facilitate deeper self-discovery. To explore their own creation, they were invited to use the first words that popped into their heads. Samuels and Lane (1998) described the healing process through words as a letter written from the heart. Words coming from deep within are released into the outside world.

May (woman, age 40) experienced calmness touching the Water. The energy of the Water filled her. She felt like she was relaxed in a tranquil lake. She picked up a Kalimba and played. She found her peace again— and much to her surprise, it was so easy. She then moved to drawing. She used both hands to touch the color paints and explored with curiosity. In the creative process, she let go of her fear and her entangled feelings. She allowed herself to release her negative emotions from deep inside. She drew a blue sky to disperse her sadness and added a flower to represent a new life. She was amazed by the true freedom in the process, the revealing power of the water, and the inspiring sounds of the Kalimba.

Ah Yuet (woman, age 34) was interested in the Metal element and experimented with the different sounds of the Metal materials, like a copper bowl and a tin lid. The sounds and tones were inspiring. She discovered her sadness of waiting for the moon. She reproduced a line from a Chinese poem "When will the bright moon come?" (明月幾時有) in her work by mixed media. She perceived the bright moon as representing good fortune. Finally she found the answer in her own creation and shared the following poem by Wang Wei:

明月松間照
清泉石上流

"Just like the moon shining through the pines and
the clear stream flowing over the rocks."

Her art revealed her positive energy, just like the moon shining through
the pines and the clear stream flowing over the rocks. The color flow on
the paper stirred her heart and made her joyous.

The feedback from the participants was encouraging. Most appreciated
the idea of integrating the Chinese concepts in expressive arts therapy.
They enjoyed using Chinese painting papers, ink, and brushes. Chinese
painting paper is soft, and good for exploring emotions. Even a single
Chinese painting brush can make various forms of strokes and facilitate
a diversity of expressions. The participants also had fun using water and
soil in exploring the inner experience. Since the materials representing
the Five Elements were new to them, they could let go of the habitual
way of doing art. This newness could facilitate spontaneous expression
and experimentation with the unknown. Each element brought out
their curiosity. Using natural objects made the art making concrete and
accessible for deeper insight.

Yin–Yang Mandala 陰陽曼佗儸

The Yin–Yang Mandala is created by blending Mandala and Yin–Yang.
Mandala is a circular form of art and a reflection of the self (Fincher,
1991). It is a sacred circle of healing, soothing, searching, experiencing,
and inspiration. Yin–Yang was mentioned in I Ching 易經 (the Book
of Changes), Chunqiu Fanlu 春秋繁露 (Rich Dew of the Spring and
Autumn Classic), Chinese cosmology, and medical theory. In Dao De
Jing 道德經, the complementarity of Yin–Yang refers to the relationship
of the male and female modes of being (Rosenlee, 2006). In Chinese
medical theory, Yin–Yang is the foundation of gendered meanings or
energy circulated in the body and the world at large. Harmony between
Yin–Yang is vital to our wellness. The Yin–Yang symbol is also round and
represents the Chinese understanding of balance. "Yin" can be our shadow,
the feminine and the unconscious of the human psyche. "Yang" represents
light, the masculine and the conscious self (Jung, 1978; Rosenlee, 2006).
By introducing arts in the Yin–Yang Mandala, we make a circular form of
visual art to represent the "Yin" and "Yang" parts.

The objectives of the "Yin–Yang Mandala" workshop were:

1. to contain the polarity in one's psyche

2. to explore and identify a potential for change and transformation

3. to attain a feeling of soothing and wholeness.

We start by making the Yin–Yang Mandala with art materials and explore it using another art modality. Sometimes we move through even more modalities. Each modality carries a unique therapeutic effect and emotive quality for the individual. Through art making, creating, moving, sounding, acting, interacting, improvising, and playing, we explore the Mandala in a holistic way. The creative exploration is action-based and process-focused. Different non-verbal media like colors, images, gesture, facial expression, voices, and words are used to explore the polarities inside oneself. The participants can experience sensory and kinesthetic stimulation in the creative healing arena. Their deeper feelings and inner struggles are visualized by creative language and artistic metaphors. With proper release of negative energy and increased self-awareness, they can integrate the Yin–Yang parts into their true selves. The Yin–Yang Mandala can also be a symbol for meditation, affirmation, and healing.

First, I invited the participants to warm up by drawing circles. They drew imaginary circles using different parts of their body, like the head, shoulders, hands, hips, and legs, after dipping into an imaginary palette. They could choose their favorite colors and stretch their bodies with all their might. They then moved freely to feel the Yin–Yang energy of their own Mandala. There is no right or wrong way. Staying still is also a movement. They were allowed to move and make sounds in any way they felt like, with safety being the only rule. They could choose to keep their eyes closed or open. It was a special experience when they focused on the inside and let their bodies take the lead. The movement led them into the meditative space where they met their own Yin–Yang. After the movements, they created their Mandala in visual art form. They chose their colors and forms by intuition.

Lai (woman, age 55) intended to draw a colorful flower to represent her feminine self (Figure 18.2). She enjoyed the feminine energy with the breezy floating fabrics in her movements. She recognized her soft and delicate sides. She hoped to keep her life blossoming, like this flower with its rich layers of colors. She felt fulfilled. I held up her Mandala and rotated it clockwise, so that she could explore her images from different perspectives. Suddenly the flower became a rotary blade—an ancient vicious weapon. This observation stunned her. It was a reflection of herself in her marriage. She yearned for a closer relationship, but she easily lost her patience and became an irritant to her husband. Looking at her Mandala, she realized how her husband felt when hit by the blade. She was acutely aware of the need to change to improve the marital relationship.

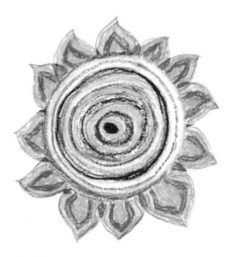

Figure 18.2 *Mandala wheel*

In a training group, Yan (woman, age 30) created a Mandala painting (Figure 18.3) about the struggle between the mind and the heart. The green heart shape (top) symbolized her heart yearning for inner peace. The black (bottom) was the messy part of her mind. It made her crazy. Between the mess and the heart, she put a yellow line representing knowledge. She hoped that knowledge could make a sensible separation protecting the heart from the mess. She further explored her Mandala through other art forms. She chose three participants from the group to represent her Heart, Knowledge, and Messy (Figure 18.4). She assigned each of them one musical instrument to make a five-minute improvisation. She watched by the side. It was interesting that Messy was strongly led by Knowledge. As Knowledge (chime) was getting louder and louder, it stimulated a strong reaction from Messy (rattle). It seemed that Messy was fighting back. When Knowledge became quieter, Heart (brass bell) and Messy changed into a duet. The improvisation truly reflected her situation. Too much knowledge only scared and confused her. She had to learn how to filter the information and listen to her true needs.

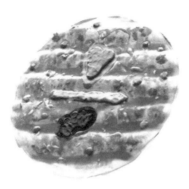

Figure 18.3 *Mandala Mind Heart*

The application of expressive arts in the Yin–Yang Mandala is based on the belief that the process can elevate our polarity from the unconscious level to the conscious level. Like Yin and Yang, the two extremities are, at the same time, complementary to each other. The therapist supports the process through full presence, empathetic understanding, and an accepting attitude. The healing process is a self-discovery journey of doing, making, visualizing, thinking, improvising, witnessing, and experiencing. From expression and exploration to awareness, the group is empowered and transformed. They are the masters of their own creative healing process. Some participants found the Yin–Yang balance between light and shadow. Some felt the harmony between feminine and masculine. Some shared that the unknown becomes known. The higher consciousness, the positive change, and the vital revolution resulted in a self-directed flow of healing. To sustain the change, they could continue the creative healing process for self-awareness, soul nourishment, and maintenance of wellness in their daily life.

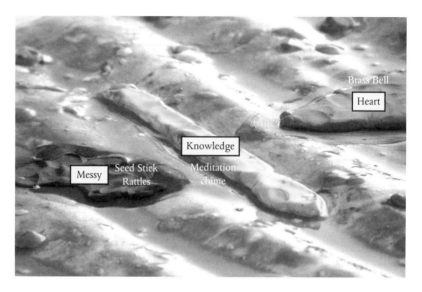

Figure 18.4 *Mandala Mind Heart music*

"Xinjie" 心結 — "Knots in the Heart"

In the Chinese language, "Xinjie" refers to knots in our heart. The knot is an analogy of suppressed and unresolved business in our heart. These knots can be guilt, shame, fear, frustration, anger, or worries. When we cannot cope with these psychological weeds, they become knots in our hearts and make us uncomfortable. To resolve these struggles, we need to come face to face with them. Then we can release them and free ourselves. In the Chinese character "jie" 結, one side, "糸," represents the silk string and the other side, "吉," means good luck. From this meaning, not all knots are bad. Knots are tied in a string to strengthen the string. We can use the knot to symbolize, record, and preserve our strengths.

The objectives are:

1. to explore our strength and weakness by making knots

2. to understand and remove the inhibitions in our inner avenue through the expressive arts

3. to identify personal resources and affirm our strengths.

I began with two warm-up activities. The first was spontaneous movements to music, which was followed by a museum pose—a freeze-frame of "here-and-now." They used percussion instruments to express their "heart" beats. Then the participants used colorful twine strings and found materials to make various assemblies of knots. Marbles, rocks, dried shells, leaves and flowers, charcoal, and egg shells are wonderful found materials. McNiff (2009) shared that it is helpful to liberate expression and generate feelings through intense concentration of an external object. In the process of exploring the objects for the knot making, we pay attention to the colors, forms, texture, and characteristics of each material. Each knot can represent strength, resources, inhibition, and limitation in life. When the knots were done, the participants had a dialogue with each knot and wrote about it. They shared with a partner or with the group. The closing ritual was an enacted play of cooking a pot of Chinese-style soup for healing. One ingredient can represent one positive trait. Each is then thrown into the pot. The soup is made of all the positive traits. The soup is "scooped" up with hands and consumed, enabling all to have a taste of the "good stuff." One can save some of the soup in one's heart as a reserve for the future.

The participants went into their own space to create, let go, and heal. I intended to observe them in a corner to minimize the disturbance to their process. It was amazing to witness how they expressed their struggles. All had their unique ways of knot making to expel inhibition and access their inner essence. Some used the knots to hide their secrets. Some projected their burdens onto the found materials and transferred their burden to the knots. Some created the knots to represent their struggle and then found ways to untie them. Some, having untied one knot, found it easy to untie the rest. Untying could be difficult, but it only reflected the reality of life. And when a knot could not be untied, staying away from it also helped. Accepting the presence of untied knots was a way of coping. Acceptance is an enactment of forgiving. By "communicating" with each knot, they gain insight and understand themselves.

Wincy (woman, age 44) felt that the knots of cancer filled her life. She was overwhelmed by low esteem, her fear of death, and an unknown emotion. She used laundry clips to represent the knots. Her whole body was entangled in clips. She felt suffocated and in pain. She realized her longing for relief and freedom. She removed and threw away these clips. I was touched.

Macy (woman, age 53) enjoyed the process of embracing her strengths. Through each knot she could visualize her unique strength. She felt her confidence when her strengths became tangible. Each knot also opened a secret doorway to her creativity, harmony, and life force. In the process of exploring the knots, she found joy in self-discovery and affirmed the beauty of her existence. She appreciated the authentic expression of feelings, insight stimulation, open communication, and heartfelt group support.

Heider (1985) shared that the person who is down-to-earth can complete a task more effectively than the person who is always side-tracked. So when the participants were mindful and attentive to the process, they could witness more clearly the possibilities in the expressive arts wellspring. They could understand their shadow, let go of the unresolved business, accept whatever emerges in life, and see the light.

Reflection

C. Rogers (cited in Rogers, 1993) emphasized the role of the therapist as being genuine, empathic, honest, congruent, and caring. His humanistic view of the true being of the therapist echoes the Confucius concept of humaneness (仁 rén). Both theories are based on empathy. Jung (1978) shared an inspiring saying by an ancient Chinese adept—"If the wrong man uses the right means, the right means works in the wrong way" (p.6). He added, "The method is merely the path, the direction taken by a man; the way he acts is the true expression of his nature." All of these concepts capture the essence of the true being of the therapist and affirm my belief in the use of self in helping others. Use of self is always an art in expressive arts therapy. It is important to use our "whole person" to be with the individuals in the creative helping process. Apart from accredited training, clinical supervision, and self-reflection, it is important to have regular hands-on arts practice to understand ourselves in a rigorous but creative way.

As we believe in the ability of individuals to create and then heal themselves, we use the arts only as a conscious process of empowerment and transformation. Each individual has a profound self-healing capacity. We have to be sensitive and mindful of our interconnectedness with each individual. We should go according to their pace and in their direction. My personal and professional experience affirms that the use of arts in a person-centered climate can achieve all these. When the therapist and the individual are on an equal footing in the healing process, the individual is no longer a recipient but a self-directed person with dignity, satisfaction and creativity.

Every community has its unique culture and language. People vary, not only in abilities and needs, but also in styles of expression and choice of art modalities. It is important to respect the culture and traditional values. I encourage people to use their native arts, familiar tools, and available materials in the creative process. Using available materials is vital in sustaining the use of arts after therapy. To understand their creative expression, I listen with curiosity, full presence, openness, and acceptance. The therapeutic process is free from diagnosis, judgment, and interpretation.

Conclusion

Corey and Corey (1987) remind us of becoming aware of our own culture and open to different cultures. Hong Kong is unique in that we have both East and West. To help firmly plant expressive arts therapy locally, the East–West difference and similarity should be utilized to create a synergy. One needs to know both cultures and amalgamate both into one entity. Chinese and local cultures, beliefs, art forms, and metaphors should be blended with expressive arts therapy and turned into a local recipe.

References

Cheng, G.M. (2000) *The Impact of Harmony on Chinese Conflict Management*. Paper presented at the Annual Meeting of the National Communication Association, 9–12 November 2000, Seattle, WA.

Corey, M. and Corey, G. (1987) *Group Process and Practice*. Pacific Grove, CA: Brooks/Cole Publishing Company.

Fincher, S.F. (1991) *Creating Mandalas for Insight, Healing, and Self-Expression*. Boston and London: Shambhala.

Heider, J. (1985) *The Tao of Leadership: Lao Tzu's Tao Te Ching Adapted for a New Age*. Atlanta, GA: Humanics.

Jung, G.C. (1978) *Jung Psychology and the East*. Princeton: Princeton University Press.

Levitt, S. (2000) *Taoist Feng Shui: The Ancient Roots of the Chinese Art of Placement*. Rochester, VT: Destiny Books.

Malchiodi, C.A. (ed.) (2005) *Expressive Therapies*. New York, NY: Guilford Press.

McNiff, S. (1981) *The Arts and Psychotherapy*. Springfield, IL: Charles Thomas.

McNiff, S. (2009) *Integrating the Arts in Therapy: History, Theory, and Practice*. Springfield, IL: Charles Thomas.

Moon, C.H. (2010) *Materials and Media in Art Therapy: Critical Understandings of Diverse Artistic Vocabularies*. London and New York: Routledge.

Mortenson, S.T. (1999) *Cultural Variations in Emotion and Effective Emotional Support Processes: Documenting Differences in the Experience, Expression, and Management of Emotional Distress*. Thesis, Purdue University.

Rappaport, L. (2009) *Focusing-Oriented Art Therapy: Accessing the Body's Wisdom and Creative Intelligence*. London: Jessica Kingsley Publishers.

Rogers, N. (1993) *The Creative Connection®: Expressive Arts as Healing*. Palo Alto, CA: Science and Behavior Books.

Rosenlee, L.H.L. (2006) *Confucianism and Women: A Philosophical Interpretation.* Albany, NY: State University of New York Press.

Rossi, E., Caretto, L. and Scheid, V. (2007) *Shen: Psycho-Emotional Aspects of Chinese Medicine.* Edinburgh: Churchill Livingstone Elsevier.

Samuels, M. and Lane, M.R. (1998) *Creative Healing: How to Heal Yourself by Tapping Your Hidden Creativity.* San Francisco, CA: Harper.

PART 6

Looking at Contemporary Asia

Chapter 19

Art Therapy and Disaster Relief in the Philippines

Gina A. Alfonso and Julia Gentleman Byers

This chapter focuses on an art therapy crisis intervention initiative in Bicol, the Republic of the Philippines (RP), following the aftermath of the typhoon and mudslide disaster killing 1000 people in November 2006. In early January 2007, barely two months after typhoon "Reming" swept the Bicol region, we had the opportunity to become firsthand witnesses to the indigenous wisdom and strength of Filipinos. The Bicolanos, the fifth largest cultural-linguistic group in the RP, are locals to Bicol, home of Mt. Mayon, the most active volcano in the country. True to the core value of Filipino personhood—*kapwa* (shared self/shared identity)— Ateneo de Naga University (AdNU) psychologists, social workers, and administrators welcomed us, an ex-patriot female Filipino and a white foreign woman (de Guia, 2005). We offered to support their rehabilitative work through humanitarian arts therapy training workshops and direct aid. Workshops conducted in three phases provided approximately 400 mudslide survivors with the space to remember and express their indigenous wisdom, resilience, and hope amidst the rubble.

The Philippine context

Filipinos, by nature, are a collectively resilient people (Tadem, 2009). Many who argue that Filipino resilience is a natural consequence of their chronic exposure to both natural and man-made (political) catastrophes emphasize the need for Filipinos to be more proactively resistant to hardships (de Quiros, 2009). Due to the geographic location of the Philippines along the Pacific Rim of Fire, however, consequential natural disasters seem to have shaped the Filipinos' psyche.

Pre-colonial Filipinos had an inherent sensitivity to natural phenomena, which ultimately governed their economic lives. Each *barangay* (community) was led by a "chief" or "council of elders," who could read the position of the moon and the stars and predict whether the coming year would be beneficial to their crops, or whether something hazardous was forthcoming. Their understanding of star constellations and sea winds also provided them with information regarding when best to navigate the sea and gave them an intimate knowledge of it (Nadeau, 2008). Collaborative ways of responding to natural calamities evolved, such as the entire village coming together to carry a house under construction to a different location during a rainstorm. Inherent in this community effort called *bayanihan* (spirit of unity to achieve a common objective) are the Filipino values identified by Enriquez (1992) of *kapwa* (shared identity, in Tagalog), *pakiramdam* (shared inner perception), and *kagandahang-loob* (shared humanity). Pakiramdam is a deep inner feeling that triggers spontaneous voluntary actions that come with a sharing of self (de Guia, 2005).

The apparent ability of present-day Filipinos to navigate repeated exposure to impose cultural, socio-political, and physical changes in their homeland somehow reflects the same resilience, creative spirituality, and problem-solving capabilities that forewarned their ancestors. Other tangible consequences to their chronic and repeated exposure to tragedy are several collective defenses that permeate daily living in the Philippines. One of these is their ability to smile through pain. Known as the people from the Land of Smiles, Filipinos are characterized as a friendly, open, and spiritual people despite their constant exposure to strife. *Bahala na* ("come what may" or "leave it to God"), another attitude stereotypically used to describe a Filipino's response to challenges, is born out of their need to make do with existing resources, often scarce, amidst the high incidence of poverty. It has its roots in the core value kapwa, which thrives on connectedness—"of man with man, of man with nature, and of man with the unseen spirit worlds, and ultimately, of man with God" (de Guia, 2007, p.3).

"Smiling and often times joking through the pain" and bahala na may be described as a sense of abandonment or surrender, springing from an underlying trust and quiet confidence and faith in God. While these seemingly escapist responses to pain may stereotypically be perceived as weaknesses, their deeper underpinnings speak to the Filipino wisdom and values embedded in their indigenous past. This continues today to carry them towards a positive vision of the future.

Rehabilitative disaster responses in the Philippines

In 2010 the Philippines ranked first worldwide among countries most affected by natural disasters (See, 2010). The Bicol region alone experiences an average of 20 to 24 natural disasters annually. Needless to say, it has been imperative that the development of effective disaster management systems remains a priority of the national government.

Disaster management has evolved through several presidential decrees since 1947. In 1978, Presidential Decree #1566 declared the National Disaster Coordinating Council (NDCC) the highest policy-making body on disaster matters in the country. It continues to be the primary coordinating council that ensures disaster preparedness, prevention, mitigation, and responses in the country.

The Department of Social Welfare and Development (DSWD), also active in disaster rehabilitation, offers play therapy as a standard service to treat traumatized children. Carandang (1987), a native Filipino and psychologist, first introduced this therapeutic intervention to local practitioners in her book *Filipino Children Under Stress*. She and her team of clinicians have conducted numerous workshops for the DSWD on the use of play therapy to treat various issues including psychological trauma (Carandang, 2009). In addition to play therapy, art therapy has recently become a burgeoning field in the country. Currently, there are a handful of Filipino art therapists trained and registered in the United States and Europe.

The C.H.ARTS framework

We based our work on Collective Healing through the Arts (C.H.ARTS), a framework we developed from various resources to serve as a process guide for each of the workshops. C.H.ARTS is a strength-based, art-centered, brief crisis intervention model with three main goals toward healing from psychological trauma caused by natural or man-made disasters:

1. *The rediscovery of collective strength and resilience.* Within a safe community, facilitators recall the survivors' historical antecedents, and form a collective narrative from which to draw collective wisdom, strength, and resilience.

2. *Self-awareness of physiological reactions associated with the traumatic event.* Understanding current (post-trauma) physical self-experience to learn self-regulation through practicing body-centered activities and engaging physically with the environment with a sense of mastery and equilibrium (Van der Kolk, 2006).

3. *The internal reframing of emotions associated with the traumatic event.* Reframing the incident by externalizing the personal narrative in a safe environment with witnesses, which allows for the careful, mindful recovery and reconstruction of oneself in relation to the experience to dissolve its continued random interference in day-to-day life (Van der Kolk, 2006).

The succeeding steps (H.E.A.L.I.N.G.) are guidelines to provide a starting point from which facilitators can develop a flow of appropriate activities and choice of materials to provide a transformative pathway from grief to the beginnings of growth.

1. H: *HONOR HISTORY*

Review literature and respectfully interview locals to recollect the history and natural collective defenses of the community and country through a thorough understanding of the culture's history of dealing with disasters.

2. E: *ESTABLISH A SENSE OF SAFETY*

Compassionately empower the participants with knowledge about the universal responses to trauma without minimizing their experience. This step develops a sense of normality and creates a container of safety and understanding, establishing trust between survivors and facilitators.

3. A: *ART THERAPY INTERVENTION*

Assess and re-assess the appropriateness of planned activities based on historical, cultural, and symptomatic data gathered. Develop culturally sensitive therapeutic art activities and art materials for the group's expression of feelings and the deeper exploration of identified psycho-emotional responses to disaster. Interweave appropriate, non-threatening, body-centered activities that help develop self-awareness leading to physical and emotional self-regulation.

4. L: *Listen*

Lay out the images for the quiet and respectful witnessing of the externalized traumatic event. Encourage a deep attending and listening to each other's narratives. Mirror back common threads in their narratives from which survivors can draw a sense of oneness and strength. Invite the group to share any physiological responses that surfaced during the creation and witnessing of artwork.

5. I: *Internal reframing*

Once grief has been externalized and processed, introduce an art process that allows survivors to retell their narratives with their desired ending. This opportunity to externally manipulate the event will help them internally reframe the experience, and regulate their emotional distress. When their images are complete, invite them individually to create a movement or series of movements in response to the art.

6. N: *Narrate*

Allow for the narration and re-narration (by a facilitator) of the new stories (through art and movement). This sharing in the context of the community offers some closure, and the regaining of a sense of control through personal agency.

7. G: *Growth*

Facilitate an artistic process where survivors can begin to discover their power to choose living over not living and to thriving through the use of positive defense mechanisms. Help them identify specific pathways to emotional self-regulation, wellness, and growth.

This framework is premised on Van der Kolk's (2006) neuropsychology research indicating that trauma treatment is most effective when emphasis is made on focusing on two aspects of an individual's experience: her *personal narrative* and its *meaning*, and her current *physiological states and action tendencies* evident in her breath, gestures, sensory perceptions, movement, emotion, and thought. Some approaches that are seen to be effective involve addressing awareness of internal sensations and physical action patterns. Mindfulness, dialectical behavior therapy, body–mind centering, yoga, and other approaches that integrate sensation and movement are some examples, to name a few. As we have observed in our own clinical work, the sensory-motor involvement in expressive art therapeutic activities can trigger sensory memories, helping individuals externalize the traumatic event subconsciously and physically. This helps reframe the internal experience by creating a new story reflecting opportunity and hope.

The case of Typhoon Reming

On 30 November 2006, Typhoon Reming caused the most severe damage in the province of Albay in the Bicol region, with almost 99 percent of the barangays affected. According to rescuers, many of those killed lived in communities at the foot of Mayon Volcano. Thus, entire villages lay buried beneath its thick, black volcanic sludge, prompting Bicol's officials to create a mass grave to avert the possibility of an epidemic resulting from the high death toll (Conde, 2006).

The severity of the devastation made the delivery of social services to survivors a logistical nightmare. The lingering stench from the corpses of the dead made the need for rehabilitative services imminent. The Center for Psychological Services of AdNU, located in Camarines Sur (next to the province of Albay), took the lead in providing mental health and social workers from various organizations with opportunities for training in psychological debriefing and trauma management. A few weeks later, we arrived at the scene and were welcomed as short-term members of the team. To aid in the acute situation, we offered alternative treatments, specifically the use of brief art therapy interventions, to help process some of the survivors' psychological traumas.

The art therapy intervention

The intervention took place in three phases over four days. Phase I involved the two-day train-the-trainers workshop. The subsequent days included Phases II and III, which included visits to Barangay Punta Tarawal and Aquinas University of Legazpi City, respectively.

Pre-workshop preparations

AdNU conducted a post-typhoon impact assessment in the provinces of Camarines Sur and Albay, where Naga City and Legazpi City are located, respectively. Based on assessment results, 400 survivors in three areas were identified to be among the 4000 at risk of severe psychological trauma. To address the shortage of trained mental health professionals and the effects of the vicious disaster, we collaborated with AdNU's team of mental health clinicians to conduct a trainer's training workshop for 51 volunteer relief workers. These trained workers were disaster survivors who were not in critical condition. The two-day crisis intervention training for volunteer workers focused on how to build and recognize art making as a tool for expression and healing. It was designed in preparation for two other on-site interventions for survivors directly affected by the mudslides. Approximately half of the group from this train-the-trainers workshop then traveled with the lead facilitators to work with survivors directly affected by the mudslides in Punta Tarawal, a coastal community severely damaged by the storm, and Aquinas University of Legazpi City (AUL), a campus almost entirely submerged in mud located two hours away from Naga City.

Phase I: Training the trainers

Together with clinical and social psychologists from AdNU, we facilitated Phase I. The collectively identified goals by the volunteer relief workers were to learn how to use the expressive arts to manage their own trauma symptoms, through the creative sharing of narratives, and to prepare to co-facilitate Phases II and III.

The flow of the workshop on both days included an interweaving of art-making and body-centered activities to allow for the collective and individual expression of hurts and hopes with the use of indigenous and traditional art materials. The last art activity of the workshop illustrates the six-step H.E.A.L.I.N.G. process indentified in the C.H.ARTS framework. Its goal was to provide the volunteer relief workers with the opportunity to express their authentic feelings approaching the daunting task of rehabilitation, and to personally experience a process they would replicate in succeeding days. The instruction for this part of the workshop was to develop a fairy tale in images using the available art materials.

While most in the group worked individually, two volunteer relief workers paired up to create a single story depicted in ten separate drawings. When all had finished their creations, we processed the pair's ten images, which they were asked to lay out on the floor. The rest of the group stood around the pictures and were invited to reflect on the beginning, middle, and end elements of the story.

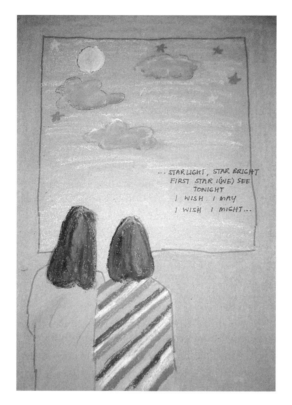

Figure 19.1 *Twinkle and Star*

Figure 19.1, the first picture in a series, displayed two friends named Twinkle and Star, watching the night sky on a journey in search for stars beyond the clouds. We invited the listeners to notice and honor the uniqueness of Twinkle and Star's friendship and ongoing loyalty. This recognition of *kapwa* (shared identity) and *pakikisama* (companionship/ esteem) as a collective strength was a way of honoring their culture and history as a people, and establishing a sense of safety for the authors of Twinkle and Star. As the process of storytelling ensued, the subsequent pictures depicted the distraught faces of Twinkle and Star as they walked through a dark black pathway. Stars were nowhere in sight. "But they have each other to hold on to" was written beneath the illustration. As Twinkle and Star continued on their journey, a star began to emerge from behind a mountain, but transformed into a larger solid sphere. This image demonstrated an internal re-framing of the emotional experience. In Picture 9, the words "And they continue to search for it…" were written. The final image, Picture 10, depicted a green seedpod (the star transformed into a sphere) lying on the black earth seeming to reveal a sense of renewed growth.

The artists of Twinkle and Star initially thought they had created a story that had nothing to do with the mudslide disaster, but the story seemed to match the entire group's current journey. This resulted in an instantaneous cathartic sigh let out by all. They seemed astonished to witness how the drawings revealed the unconscious projection of the mudslide disaster and the emergence of the people's core values and resilience in response to the situation.

Enriquez (1992) and de Guia (2005), experts on *Pagkataong Filipino* (Value System of Philippine Psychology), identified kapwa to be at its core, but included other values such as pakikisama, *lakas-ng-loob* (guts), *kalayaan* (freedom), and *karangalan* (dignity) also apparent in the story of Twinkle and Star and other narratives in workshop phases II and III. The beginning of the story of Twinkle and Star was marked by an attempt to reframe the event and to literally reflect hope, possibly through the image of the star. It was characterized also by a sense of unity or kapwa. Toward the middle of the story, as the loss in physical surroundings was apparent, Twinkle and Star continued on their journey, but were smiling through their pain. They continued to plod through the mud and resolved to help their compatriots make meaning out of their pain (lakas-ng-loob). This led up to the end, where the experience of growth seemed to be represented by the seedpod sprouting out of the black earth (kalayaan).

Other forms of creative and emotional work were found in the metaphoric use of materials in the art created throughout the workshop. The gauge, tension, and strength of string, tape, and other binding materials seemed symbolic of the way people attached to others. Individuals who were deeply traumatized and temporarily unable to join another in a shared identity revealed fragmented or overly knotted work. Other three-dimensional artwork was disorganized, chaotic, or over-compartmentalized (Byers, 2011).

Phase II: Rebuilding community through art and storytelling

The objective of this intervention was to honor the narratives of Barangay Punta Tarawal survivors, whose homes had been buried. This brief community-based workshop was led by the team of core and volunteer facilitators. It was conducted in the partly devastated Barangay public elementary school, accessible only by boat. Traditional art materials were used such as paper, crayons, markers, plasticine, and wire.

The workshop began with all children and adult survivors, gathered in a circle, singing and engaging in movement. The large group then broke off into groups of three led by one facilitator. Survivors introduced themselves and then created stories in images with the available materials. The facilitators replicated their experience in Phase I and each survivor was to create his or her own fairy tale. These stories were documented in writing and honored within the group.

As the small groups came together for the final activity, an elderly woman wanted to share the story of her grief over the loss of her family. Spontaneously, other survivors responded with compassion and young children gathered around her to offer their support through their drawings, clay, and wire sculptures, demonstrating kagandahang-loob.

To conclude the large group process, Julia narrated a Filipino story about *Lola* (grandmother), a mythical tale of an elderly woman whose magic powers allowed her hair to grow long enough to entwine and keep safe all the people from a great typhoon. As the rest of the group listened, they were invited to create symbolic sculptures with wire, which they interconnected to form a protective shield like Lola's hair. The participants, all survivors of the devastating typhoon, were encouraged to keep their creations as remembrances of their collective resilience and strength, and their connectivity as members of one community (kapwa).

Phase III: Rediscovering collective strengths through art

Approximately 17 volunteer relief workers from Phase I accompanied us to Aquinas University in Legazpi City. The facilitating team had only three hours for this workshop with 171 mudslide survivor participants. The process began in a large group format, with an opening song and movement exercises, followed by small group work. Each cluster was invited to use the available mixed media materials to capture the experience of their current realities. Traditional art materials such as paint, glue, wire, markers, crayons, and plasticine were used along with other indigenous materials such as twigs, leaves, and straw.

After all three-dimensional group art pieces were complete, the participants were asked to leave their poster-size images on the floor while they engaged in a witnessing of each other's artwork in silence. Later, they were invited to share their own narratives. The emergent themes that surfaced were those of pain, perseverance as a community (kapwa), and hope. The themes of hope and growth appropriately paved the way for the final activity where the community set collective and individual goals for rebuilding their campus and their lives with dignity (karangalan) beyond the existing devastation.

Before Phase III began, we explored the art media available and noticed that the university had prepared earthenware terracotta clay as a primary art supply. Upon seeing this, we approached the host team to explain how the physical properties of the loose, wet clay were almost identical to the physical properties of the mud that had figured so prominently in the disaster. We were concerned that the use of such a medium so early in the acute traumatic responses could bring up highly regressive experiences, opening up deep and intense feelings of grief, anger, and desperation that may not be contained within the time restrictions of the workshop. Given the brief intervention, we felt that people might feel a more appropriate sense of control through using materials that had a bit more structure and resilience. In addition, the logistics of using wet clay with no appropriate clean-up facilities was problematic. The wet clay was replaced with modeling clay, wire, and straws.

Discussion

Throughout Phases I, II, and III, the survivors' collective defenses were apparent particularly as we began each workshop. Smiles were as abundant as the mud surrounding the areas we visited. As humanitarian art therapists, we approached the mission with a focus on preserving and restoring continuities at the individual, family, organizational, and community levels, and on mobilizing collective strengths and skills (Omer and Alon, 1994). Being outsiders, we did not approach the work with the desire to inform another culture about how to proceed, but were there as witnesses to their concrete expressions of pain and hope through art. Storytelling through art allowed us to connect with each survivor beyond language through a shared inner perception (pakiramdam). Ironically, the very survivors' shared humanity (kapwa) and generosity of spirit (kagandahang-loob), evident as they welcomed us, made meeting them in their pain and their shared sense of hope instantaneous and life-changing. This very experience mirrored the indigenous Filipino core values.

Results of our post-intervention assessment revealed the common themes of a shared identity as survivors, resilience, and growth throughout the three phases. These values offered a starting point from which the survivors could begin the process of continuing to function, to build a new history, and to strengthen interpersonal bonds beyond the tragedy.

Another unanimous observation was the spirit of hope permeating through their smiling defenses evident even in the images they created. The survivors consistently showed up for the sessions with a spontaneous openness to life. Their strong sense of spirituality was reflected in their lightness of spirit despite the heaviness of their situation. Along with the smiles, we were particularly aware of the importance of paying attention to signs of vicarious trauma and compassion fatigue. Debriefing after the workshop was necessary for the management of all volunteer relief workers' and our own symptoms.

Implications

Based on this experience, we noted several factors that may be applicable to practicing art therapy as a rehabilitative response to other disaster-prone areas in Asia. A very close collaboration with the local host team in designing the process flow and deciding on the materials to be used is essential. A sense of openness and resilience to the possibility of time constraints, physical challenges, and a sudden change in the number of participants is also of importance. Another key factor is the benefit of beginning with a trainer's training workshop to multiply the number of relief workers and to facilitate greater access to appropriate rehabilitative services. Play and art therapy responses were effectively used in this case with up to 400 participants in four days due to the initial training with volunteer relief workers. Therapeutic art activities learned from Phase I were also echoed to other volunteer relief workers unable to attend the trainer's training. Finally, a non-negotiable factor for a rehabilitative intervention to be successful is the establishment of trust between facilitators and participants, even if it can sometimes be challenging, albeit possible, in short-term work. In this case, we aimed to consciously stay attuned to the need to create a healthy holding space for all. Finally, to ensure a healing environment, it is necessary to keep mindful of self-care. Facilitators also need to lean on each other. This could model to participants the importance of mutual support in challenging times.

Conclusion

In the case of the Filipinos, their indigenous wisdom, inherent collective resilience, and strength as a people are evident across the entire gamut of their experiences from the pre-colonial times to the present, especially in the most poverty and disaster-stricken areas, such as the Bicol region. This important piece of information allowed the facilitators to create a healthy and safe holding space for healing to take place, and helped them build on the Bicolanos' ability to transition from a state of desolation to feelings of hope. The art process and artwork produced affirmed and captured this concretely. It was evident that the creative process mimicked the participants' ability to transition gently from a state of grief to consolation, eventually turning their crisis into renewed growth and opportunity.

Acknowledgements

We would like to offer our sincerest thanks to Fr. Joel Tabora, President of AdNU in 2007, and Dr. Ruffy Ramos III, Full Professor and Counseling Psychologist at AdNU, for giving us the opportunity to work, learn, and heal with the AdNU Counseling Center's Team, volunteers, and the communities affected by the devastation caused by Typhoon Reming.

References

Byers, J. (2011) Article 50. "Humanitarian art therapy and mental health counseling." *Vistas 2011*. Available at http://counselingoutfitters.com/vistas/vistas_2011_TOC-section_09.htm, accessed on 8 February 2012.

Carandang, M.L. (1987) *Filipino Children Under Stress: Family Dynamics and Therapy*. Loyola Heights, Quezon City: Ateneo de Manila University Press.

Carandang, M.L. (2009) *The Magic of Play: Children Heal Through Art Therapy*. Pasig City, Philippines: Anvil Publishing.

Conde, C.H. (2006) "Typhoon Durian triggers landslides in the Philippines." *The New York Times*, 1 December. Available at www.nytimes.com/2006/12/01/world/asia/01iht-phils.3744640.html, accessed on 4 November 2011.

de Guia, K. (2005) *Kapwa: The Self in the Other, Worldviews and Lifestyles of Filipino Culture-Bearers*. Pasig City, Philippines: Anvil.

de Guia, K. (2007) "Indigenous Filipino values: A foundation for a culture of non-violence." *Towards a Culture of Nonviolence*. Available at www.ugnayan.110mb.com/public_html/cnv%20stories/Indigenous%20Values.html, accessed on 4 November 2011.

de Quiros, C. (2009) "Filipino resilience." *Philippines: Philippine Daily Inquirer*. Available at http://opinion.inquirer.net/inquireropinion/columns/view/20091020-231079/Filipino-resilience, accessed on 4 November 2011.

Enriquez, V. (1992) *From Colonial to Liberation Psychology*. Quezon City, Philippines: University of the Philippines Press.

Nadeau, K. (2008) *The History of the Philippines (The Greenwood Histories of the Modern Nations)*. Westport, CT: Greenwood.

Omer, H. and Alon, N. (1994) "The continuity principle: A modified approach to disaster and trauma." *American Journal of Community Psychology 22*, 2, 273–287.

See, D. (2010) *RP World's Most Disaster-Prone – Study.* Philippines: Manila Bulletin. Available at www.mb.com.ph/articles/271081/rp-world-s-most-disasterprone-study, accessed on 4 November 2011.

Tadem, E. (2009) "The Filipino peasant in the modern world: Tradition, change and resilience." *Philippine Political Science Journal 30*, 53.

Van der Kolk, B.A. (2006) "Clinical implications of neuroscience research in PTSD." *Annals of the New York Academy of Sciences 1071*, 277–293.

Chapter 20

Surviving Shame

Engaging Art Therapy with Trafficked Survivors in South East Asia

Lydia Atira Tan

Human trafficking is the illegal trade of human beings through abduction, threat or force, deception, fraud, or "sale" for the purposes of sexual exploitation, forced labor, servitude, or slavery, especially of women and children. In Cambodia, where most of the population live in economic hardship and are subjected to gender disparity, an influx of vulnerable young girls and women are being trafficked internally and internationally, mostly as sex workers. In a report by the UN Inter-Agency Project on Human Trafficking (UNIAP) in 2008, trafficking in persons is the fastest growing and most lucrative form of international criminal activity. It is the world's third largest criminal activity and biggest violation of human rights (UNIAP, n.d.).

In 2005, I created an art therapy program with Agir Pour Les Femmes En Situation Precaire (AFESIP) in Cambodia, working closely with sex trafficked survivors who were undergoing rehabilitation and reintegration after repatriation from Thailand and leaving local brothels. The objectives of this program focused on supporting the healing of psychological and emotional trauma of sex trafficked survivors in the shelter, while eliciting data to assess the mental health needs of the clients. The qualitative data collected was used to lobby for effective preventative and curative national policies. This chapter will describe the process of the art therapy program and art therapy research process with the sex trafficked survivors in Cambodia. It will describe how it worked, and how art therapy helped to support the healing of sexual, psychological, physical, and emotional trauma.

Sex trafficking in Cambodia

Cambodia is a source, transit, and destination country for human trafficking. The traffickers are reportedly organized crime syndicates, parents, relatives, friends, intimate partners, and neighbors (UNIAP, n.d.). ECPAT Cambodia (n.d.), an anti-trafficking Non-Government Organization (NGO), reports that as many as one-third of the trafficking victims in prostitution are children, many of whom are as young as seven years old (Cochrane, 1998). Many women and children are internally trafficked within Cambodia from rural to urban areas for sexual exploitation. Many victims believe that they will be working as domestic servants, waitresses, and factory workers, only to be later coerced and forced into sex work (UNIAP, n.d.). There are also many Cambodian women and children who are internationally trafficked into Thailand as sex workers (Bobak, 1996).

Although poverty is the most significant cause of trafficking, UNIAP (n.d.) states that sex trafficking has increased because of a number of factors, including socio-economic imbalance between rural and urban areas, increased tourism, and a lack of employment, education, and safe migration. Victims of trafficking often come from family backgrounds of broken homes, domestic violence, alcoholism, and physical, sexual, and emotional abuse, making them easy targets for exploitation. When recruited by brokers in a village, the girls' families are told they will be employed and be able to send money home. After a girl is purchased and after her sexual encounter with her first customer, the girl is considered to be "used goods" and her value drops dramatically to as little as $2USD per sexual transaction. The enslaved girls risk abuse or must stay until their debt to their purchaser is paid off. Working off their purchase amount is difficult, if not impossible, since the owners consider the girls indebted to them for their constantly mounting expenses for food, clothing, medical expenses, and abortions. As a result, a brothel owner will hold a girl prisoner until she becomes too old or too ill to attract customers (Bobak, 1996).

In many Asian cultures, a girl has lower status than a man and is expected to serve and provide for the family. An older daughter is expected to give up her own education and future so as to provide support for her younger siblings to go to school. These women are under pressure to stay in the sex industry and work to provide as much as they can for their families. Even if by chance some may be freed, many choose to go back into those dangerous communities and dysfunctional families out of a sense of loyalty. Additionally, most of the issues that led them to being trafficked in the first place continue to exist in their communities. As a result, many are repeatedly re-trafficked by the same traffickers through shame and trickery.

Without the proper and effective long-term psychosocial care, it is difficult for a sex trafficked survivor to lead a normal life. In my years as an art therapist working with sex trafficked survivors, many of the psychological issues identified include post-traumatic stress disorder (PTSD), self-harming behaviors, suicidal thoughts, avoidance, disassociation, helplessness, border-line personality disorder, powerlessness, disturbance of memory, self-blaming, self-despising, low self-esteem, anxiety, stress, and HIV/AIDS.

Cultural conditioning and values

The culture of the Cambodian survivors is an important one to take into account. In any cross-cultural interaction with a client group, it is vital to understand their cultural beliefs and values, in this case specifically how society treats women. As mentioned before, in Cambodian society a woman is considered second-class compared with a man. The woman is in a place of servitude, constantly serving everyone else but herself. In Cambodia, alcohol and domestic violence is rife, especially in the poorer provinces of Cambodia, and women are often the victims of violence and dysfunction. Once a woman has lost her virginity, she is considered not worthy of marriage. The girl is branded as a "bad" girl, and holds a bad reputation in the community, leading to discrimination, scandal, and gossip.

Moreover, in most Asian countries, it is not culturally appropriate to express feelings of negativity, such as anger. In a hierarchical society, women are not encouraged to stand up and voice their opinion. They are expected to speak when spoken to and expected to "save face," which is not to embarrass their families. In this context, it is a taboo for the women to speak about family issues and they invariably remain silent about the fact that they were trafficked by their family members. Taking all these considerations into account, an art therapist must hold a space for the participants which is culturally sensitive, empathic, and appropriate to the context.

"The River of Life": Expressive art therapy research

The narratives of the trafficked survivors are presented from a socio-ethnographical approach (Berg, 2004). This approach focuses on using narrative analysis as a form of both research and therapy. The object of the investigation is the story itself. These case studies demonstrate the effectiveness of art therapy both as a qualitative research tool to collect and analyze the subjective psychological and emotional experiences of trafficked women, before, during, and after being sold into the sex trade, and as an effective psychological intervention.

Participants

In this Kitakyushu Forum for Asian Women (KFAW) funded research project, 12 survivors of sex trafficking from the art therapy program in AFESIP Cambodia were recruited and engaged in art therapy. The clients were girls and women aged from 16 to 28 years of age. Some of them were HIV positive, and some of them were single mothers with children. They had been living in the AFESIP Cambodia Shelter for 1–2 years, undertaking vocational training in order to be reintegrated back into Cambodian society and the community. The number of participants was kept to a minimum so as to maintain the ability to work on a very personal level within a group setting. Through artwork, creative writing, and poetry, the clients were encouraged to describe their experiences as much as possible. The work in a group served to create solidarity and a sense of community between the group members, which was an important part of the healing process.

Setting

The art therapy workshop created a psychologically safe environment in which the work could take place, which was a necessary and important factor in creating a psychological containment. The workshops took place behind a closed door, with no interruptions. In addition, the participants had a relationship of trust and rapport with the assistants and translators, as well as respect for the facilitator's non-judgmental and accepting stance. It also helped that this workshop occurred after a year of working with the art therapist. The participants felt acknowledged and valued. If the participants felt any hints of judgment or discrimination, they would be less likely to share their stories and experiences openly.

It was important also for the participants to know that the workshop would be followed up with individual art therapy and counseling. We were aware that beginning to work and research with this vulnerable population could potentially trigger feelings or memories that could feel overwhelming for the individual. By offering the possibility of individual therapy, we ensured that those who were in need of further support would have access to adequate psychological care. Another element which contributed to the support of the clients was the development of a peer group. The participants in the group were their friends in the shelter, and they were able to support each other through this process. When we began the workshops the group had already spent a few months living in the shelter with each other, so they were familiar with each other, and had established a group rapport.

Framework

The workshop was based on Morita's (2006) expressive art therapy research methodology, which allowed the workshop to serve as both art therapy and research. The steps included the following:

1. Introduce the purpose and intention to the participants.

2. Listen to the feedback and the response of the participants to the purpose and intention. Informing them of the purpose of the workshop gave the survivors a sense of meaning of their experiences and empowered them by voicing their past experiences to advocate against trafficking.

3. Facilitate the art therapy exploration and therapeutic process.

4. Invite the participants to share their work.

5. Acknowledge, appreciate, and affirm each participant's strength and openness in sharing their work. Encourage the participants to reflect on their journey and the question: What did I learn from my story?

6. Follow up the art therapy exploration with further counseling and art therapy, and an individual rehabilitation treatment plan based on the research findings and needs of the trafficked survivors.

The creative tools that were employed in this exercise were paints, oil pastels, collage, color pens, pencils, and creative writing. Large white cardboard pieces of paper (size A1) were glued together to create a big "River." It was useful to give the participants a structure of storytelling to guide and assist the clients through creative expression. By creating five images using the symbol of a river as a chronological account of their lives, the participants explored their life-stories, experiences, feelings, and situations. The images in "The River of Life" included the following:

- The first image addressed their experiences, feelings, circumstances and events in life before being trafficked.

- The second image focused on how they were being trafficked, what happened to them during this process, and their feelings towards being trafficked.

- The third image aimed at grasping their experiences and feelings about being sexually exploited and sold into sex work. They were encouraged to express the struggles and difficulties that they encountered when they were working, and their feelings and reactions of being sold.

- The fourth image captured their experience of being rescued. They were encouraged to describe how they were rescued, and to convey their feelings of being rescued.

- The fifth image expressed where they were in the present, and how they felt staying in the after-care center and their plans for the future.

The participants consciously transformed their past exploitative experiences into a positive framework and were empowered to assist and support others who had been through similar experiences of trafficking.

Process

There is a Cambodian saying: "Once a cloth is dirtied, the value is lost and we have to throw it away." These trafficked survivors believe that they are dirtied cloth, and many of them feel that they will never gain back their dignity and respect in society. Despite this strong social conditioning, and the negative connotations associated with their past, they were able to speak freely. The participants were very open and honest in sharing their stories; in fact they had begun sharing even before starting the creative process. Their willingness to risk feeling exposed and vulnerable in sharing and revealing private and painful parts of their lives despite the discrimination against them was very powerful.

Through the group process and the creation of a safe and non-judgmental environment, the women were able to gain a different perspective on their lives, a perspective where healing could be nurtured and could naturally occur. Many of the participants expressed that they felt very happy and proud about what they had achieved, and there was a sense of empowerment through the process of creation and sharing.

During the workshop, there were opportunities for the participants to share their individual stories with the facilitator while they were creating their artwork. In these sharings, the women would often express feelings and thoughts which were darker and deeper than they were able to share in a group setting. This seemed of benefit for those individuals who needed this extra support, and provided a setting in which they could express themselves outside the social context.

As an example, one participant described that she had a boyfriend whom her father rejected. She felt hurt by her father's rejection, and ran away from her home to Phnom Penh. In Phnom Penh, she met a woman who promised her a job, but sold her to a brothel instead. After working at the brothel for some time, one of her clients brought her to the police. The police, in turn, brought her to the AFESIP shelter where she has been studying sewing. Her journey is expressed in "The River of Life" (Figure 20.1).

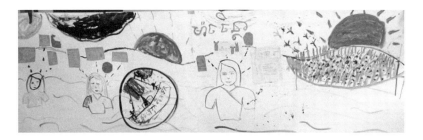

Figure 20.1 *"The River of Life"*

She drew a picture of herself being tortured and abused by the brothel owner (Figure 20.2). She is the woman on the left, and the man on the right is the owner. When she would refuse to have sex with the clients, her boss would force her to have sex through physical abuse. She used red to represent her pain. She is kneeling down in front of the man, and her eyes are black from crying. This drawing has a sense of immense pain, sadness, and shame.

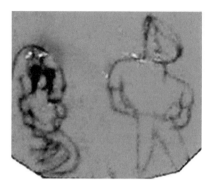

Figure 20.2 *Image of abuse*

In a later image (Figure 20.3), she drew a mandala as a collective representation of her experience of being trafficked and working as a sex worker. The figures are black in color, and there is a frantic feeling in this image of a sense of drowning. She has drawn a symbol of a boat drowning in the water. The image on the right depicts hanging herself, with a dark cloud overhead. This image symbolizes her thoughts about committing suicide to end the pain that she feels inside.

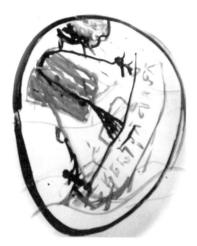

Figure 20.3 *Drowning boat*

Results

In looking at the stories that emerged, we can get insight into the details of these women's experiences.

Pre-trafficking

The pre-trafficking experience includes the following:

- Family background of poverty, lack of food, and shelter.
- Little or no education.
- Big families with many children, with the survivors being the firstborn or eldest daughter.
- Family dysfunction such as domestic violence or abuse.
- Alcoholism.
- Divorce or breakdown in family structure.
- Arguments and fights in family.
- Family expectations for the survivor to provide financially.

All of the survivors came from situations where they were vulnerable and alone. Their lack of education and life experience made them easy targets for traffickers to exploit. The themes that run through their pre-trafficking experience reflect the documented factors for sex trafficking.

Life in the brothels and experiences of being sold in the sex industry

The themes of being trafficked were the following:

- They were alone and vulnerable.
- They were manipulated into trusting the wrong person.
- They were coerced and lied to, and tortured, abused, and drugged into the sex industry.
- They had no choice but to comply.
- In the time in the brothels, they were abused physically, raped, some almost killed, and many of them were given drugs to take.

- They were not allowed to leave the brothel until they paid their debt off.
- Many of them were "rescued" from the brothels either by the police or by their clients.

In addition to these themes, they expressed the following emotions:

- depression
- helplessness
- pain
- anger
- fear
- hopelessness
- shame
- guilt
- hate (towards their perpetrators and those who exploited them)
- despair.

In the brothels, these women reported being tortured and abused physically, emotionally, psychologically, and sexually. They were given drugs and forced into the sex trade against their will. They had to serve many customers a day. Some of the younger girls were locked into a small, dark room without food and water until they complied with the wishes of the brothel owners. They all felt psychologically, and emotionally traumatized from their time in the brothels, and suffered from a range of psychological symptoms. For all of the women this was a dark and depressing time of their lives.

Post-trafficking

The themes of their post-trafficking and rehabilitation experiences were the following:

- Their need for financial independence so as to provide for their families.
- The need for a stable safe place that provided food and shelter.
- Their need for justice.

- Their dreams to lead normal lives (e.g. marriage and starting a family).
- Their desires of being happy and putting their past behind them.
- Their need to move on and integrate back in their communities.
- Their dream of being successful.
- Their dream of having a safe place they can call their own.
- The healing and support that they get from their community and new friends in the shelter.

The themes in the rehabilitation and healing after being trafficked all included their desires and need to heal from their past experiences, and to lead normal, healthy lives in the community where they would be able to support themselves and their families. All of them expressed that the community and friends that they had made in the shelter were a crucial part of healing.

Implications

"The River of Life," with its two-pronged approach, research and art therapy, helped the participants create new meaning and purpose in their stories. Prior to the workshop, their stories were shrouded in shame and guilt. However, through this process, the participants transformed their stories into a tool that could help other women who were both trafficked and as a prevention resource for women and girls who were at risk of being trafficked. This purpose and meaning created a new way of perceiving their experiences, and gave them a new sense of hope, self-confidence, and self-esteem. In a short period of time, this narrative art therapy exercise was found to be effective in depicting the survivors' stories and experiences.

Psychological benefits

Often it is difficult to find the language to describe and process traumatic experiences. Visual art allows for this expression through a non-verbal means. Traumatic experiences are encoded in non-verbal imagery and that is often difficult to verbalize because such experiences are encoded in the non-verbal imagery pathways of the mind (Breat and Ostroff, 1985). Through narrating their stories, art therapy has been an effective tool in assisting the participants in overcoming the shame and guilt that they feel, and finding words for that which is or was beyond words.

The workshop supported the survivors to reflect on their emotions and journeys from a different perspective. In art therapy, the participant obtains another perspective through their artwork, and is invited to build a relationship with the "story." The clients were able to reflect on what they learned from their experiences, their feelings, and needs so as to heal and grow. The reflection process was nurtured through a series of questions posed by the facilitator about their experiences. This process seemed to provide clarity for the participants and helped them to process the trauma and abuse. The clients seemed to gain insight and clarity into their emotions and stories through this language of symbols and images.

Additionally, many of the women began to understand that it was of no fault of their own that they were coerced and exploited into the sex industry. They realized that trafficking is an organized form of crime and that traffickers belong to massive rings that involve neighbors, families, and community. They came to see that they were naïve and vulnerable at that time with a genuine longing to serve their parents and siblings. Additionally, they acknowledged their inner strength of having survived such an ordeal.

The participants realized that they were not alone in their experiences and suffering, and felt connected with the other group members. A sense of community, solidarity, and strength was created in the group. Prior to this workshop, they felt isolated and withdrawn from society. Understanding that others felt the same way lessened the sense of isolation.

Informing intervention models

The findings from the research workshop were used to create effective individual treatment plans for each participant, by providing insight into the emotions and unresolved issues for each person. It also allowed for an understanding of the interventions that were most useful in the shelters and how to suit these to both the settings and culture. For example, the workshop led to improvements in the quality of therapeutic care of the shelter for the participants. Prior to the workshop, it took a long time for them to build up trust and rapport with each other and the caretakers in the shelter. Beyond this shelter, the themes helped to inform more effective long-term psychological curative interventions for Cambodian women nationally. Through the project, we learnt about the important therapeutic and cultural factors that are essential to take into account for future intervention models. Under the right circumstances, the expressive art therapies are effective tools of healing, helping these women to heal in a gentle and non-invasive way.

Prosecution benefits

Victims have the support to file civil suits and pursue legal action against traffickers in most anti-trafficking NGOs. Most of the time, the victim is re-traumatized through the legal process because the victim has to undergo intense questioning in the court of law against the trafficker. However, in this art therapy project, one of the participant's perpetrators was brought to justice through her artwork and stories. Her images and symbols portrayed her feelings and the psychological damage that she was subject to in a very powerful and poignant way. It was not necessary for her to testify in court against her perpetrator; her artwork and stories were considered to be enough. In this case it served to save needless re-traumatization for the survivor in the court of law, yet simultaneously supported the prosecution process.

Policy and advocacy

In the creation of curative and preventative measures and policies protecting sex trafficked survivors, the themes and qualitative data collected from this research methodology were used to advocate for the psychological and emotional support for these women. Many policy makers are not sufficiently informed about the reality and mental health issues these women face in their communities and while they are being trafficked. Through the powerful images and stories told, the policy makers are able to understand at a deeper level the psychological scars that the survivors face. With these research projects, it is possible to raise the standard of psychological care in the shelters.

The artwork that came out of the art therapy workshops, and the images and stories, were used to raise awareness and the prevention of sex trafficking nationally. The Art2Healing Project engaged in art exhibitions with AFESIP Cambodia, raising awareness about mental health issues with trafficked survivors. These exhibitions were a very powerful tool in supporting the prevention of trafficking in the community, and supporting the understanding of the psychological and emotional implications of sex trafficking.

In addition to the above, one of the objectives of this research project was to assist the process of creating effective mental health curative and preventative policies for sex trafficked survivors in Asia. The findings of this research project were presented in many anti-trafficking conferences by Dr. Akihito Morita, visiting researcher from the Kitakyushu Forum for Asian Women (KFAW). The qualitative research information was shared with other NGOs who lobby for such policies.

Conclusion

The expressive art therapy research methodology has demonstrated that it can serve as a psychological and emotional intervention for the trafficked women in Cambodia. This process has improved and empowered the life and mental health of many women by adding a sense of purpose and meaning to their lives. Through the creative process, the participants were able to process their pain and experiences in a safe environment. The qualitative information and artwork collected during the research contributed to the creation of more effective models of psychological intervention. These interventions are necessarily sensitive to the cultural context of the participants, as well as providing information for individual and personal treatment plans.

The Art2Healing Project hopes to expand the utilization of this modality further in the field of trafficking in persons in other cultural settings, and so far has developed and taught this methodology to different NGOs and governmental agencies in Cambodia, Laos PDR, and Nepal.

References

Berg, B.L. (2004) *Qualitative Research Methods*, 5th edn. Boston, MA: Pearson.

Bobak, L. (1996) "For sale: The innocence of Cambodia." *Ottawa Sun*, 24 October. Available at www.catwinternational.org/factbook/Cambodia.php, accessed on 4 November 2011.

Breat, E.A. and Ostroff, R. (1985) 'Imagery and PTSD: An overview.' *American Journal of Psychiatry 142*, 417–424.

Cochrane, J. (1998) "Child's tragedy raises profile of Rights March." *South China Morning Post*, 2 Febraury. Available at www.catwinternational.org/factbook/Cambodia.php, accessed on 4 November 2011.

ECPAT Cambodia (n.d.) ECPAT Directory: East Asia and the Pacific. Available at http://ecpat.net/Ei/Ecpat_directory.asp?id=76&groupID=3, accessed on 4 November 2011.

Morita, A. (2006) "Expressive art therapy research methodology." *Asian Breeze Magazine*, November, 6–9.

UNIAP (n.d.) Census data revisited. Cambodian Overview Population. Available at www.humantrafficking.org/countries/cambodia, accessed on 4 November 2011.

Chapter 21

The Search for Identity in Thailand

A Personal Account of Professional Art Therapy Development

Piyachat Ruengvisesh Finney

In this chapter, I review my personal process of integrating Eastern and Western values, belief systems, and the use of arts through Thai culture. I integrate my personal experience into my professional work. The process of understanding the politics of professional identity, and the struggles and challenges in finding a voice, have been a rewarding and worthwhile experience. In addition, I write about some of the clinical services and training programs that I have established and am currently expanding in Thailand.

Levels of culture

"Welcome to the Land of Smiles" is one of the first signposts you will pass as you arrive at Suvarnabhumi International Airport in Bangkok, Thailand. As we walk down the corridors to the immigration checkpoint, we are surrounded by a multi-media display of Thai cultural arts ranging from paintings of temples, water color depictions of floating markets, and huge sculptures of mythical characters. For the viewer, a sense of curiosity about this mysterious historical culture mixed with growth of Western modernization, as represented by shiny art pieces and sculptures, glare at you. With the contemporary trend of globalization and expansion of the workforce to different countries, more and more attention is being given to the subject of cross-cultural transition.

According to Pollock and Van Reken (2001):

> Learning culture is more than learning to conform to external patterns of behavior. Culture is also a system of shared assumptions, beliefs, and values. It is the framework from which we interpret and make sense of life and the world around us. (p.40)

Kohls' (as cited in Pollock and Van Reken, 2001) idea of the Cultural Iceberg is relevant to this notion of culture and its significance (Figure 21.1). He explains the concept as: "The part above the water can be identified as the *surface culture*. Underneath the water where no one can see is the *deep culture*" (p.40). To the above ideas, Pollock and Van Reken create and add a conceptual framework as illustrated by five transitional stages. I would like to demonstrate my personal process as illustrated by these five stages: involvement, leaving, transition, entering, and re-involvement.

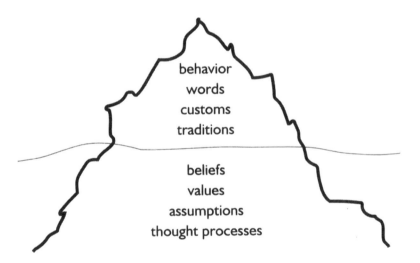

Figure 21.1 *Dr. Kohls' Cultural Iceberg*
Source: Pollock and Van Reken 2001

A personal account on the art of experience in two different worlds

My exposure to a cross-cultural environment led to my experiencing the process of assimilation and adaptation of behaviors, values, and attitudes quite early on in life.

Involvement

Throughout my primary years, I was very involved both in academic and extra-curricular activities. I had a clear role of the class leader and had a large circle of close friends. Our group always had a strong cohesion whether it was participation in sports, a debate on controversial issues, or school-related activities. After completing Prathom 7 (in the Thai educational system this is an equivalent of Grade 7 in the US system and Year 8 in the UK system), I decided to switch from a Thai to a US curriculum.

Leaving

Feeling invisible is one of the experiences Pollock and Van Reken (2001) described in this stage. Although I still lived in Thailand, I underwent a cultural adaptation in this transition. The expectations and performance within the US system are: to be assertive (both in expressing your needs and feelings as well as solving problems by confronting and negotiating, rather than being submissive and compromising); to be accountable for your actions (with courage rather than shame); and follow your dreams (be attentive to your needs, wishes, and feelings, rather than do what is good for others and suppress your needs). After a period of two years of some characteristic assimilation, I applied and was accepted into a private preparatory boarding school in Massachusetts, US. This experience was a bigger change, as now I experienced some of what Pollock and Van Reken (2001) defined as being a Third Culture Kid, which "is a person who has spent a significant part of his or her developmental years outside the parents' culture" (p.19). Leaving was sad, but it was also mixed with excitement of the new world.

Transition

The *Transition* stage of chaos at the feeling level is the next stage, and indeed it took some time before I became settled into my setting and my defined role. In the beginning I struggled with feeling that I did not fit in. Discomfort with certain Western behaviors, feeling inferior, and confusion with my identity were all in the mix of my experience of transition to the US. At the time I did not have the words to describe this alienation and sense of isolation. From high school, to college, and then to graduate school, I was busy trying to adapt without much attention to my inner process.

The acknowledgement of the transitional process (shifting from one culture to another) did not come to my attention until August 1986 when I attended a prerequisite colloquium, which was a week-long residential trip for newly admitted students to the Expressive Therapies Masters Program at Lesley College in Cambridge, MA. It was an initiation into the world of expressive therapy and experiential exercises to understand and gain insights both on the intrapsychic and interpersonal levels. In a journal entry on 17 August 1986, I wrote:

> First night, there were lots of feelings going on inside me, mainly nervousness, worrying if I could fit in... We formed a circle; then, one by one, people began to join in a chant, a way to connect and bring about group cohesion. It didn't take me long to join in... I could feel that people in our group do have respect for each other.

In another interesting entry, I wrote about a dream I expressed through an art therapy process (Figure 21.2) that led to an exploration of the unconscious mind. I wrote:

> I was in a dark, dark room listening in a storytelling workshop... Suddenly, there was a glow of fire coming into our room. It was like a big blast of fire but no sound! The fire itself was beautiful; I called it "The Magic Fire"... I found myself in another room now. There was an old friend from my high school. She handed me the broom and gestured over to two rolls of cards on the floor as if she wanted me to clean up. I went over and swept them without realizing that they were already nicely lined up side by side. "Oh no," I said, "I messed them up. Each roll (role) was already in its own group."

I woke up in horror. Could this be related to my anxiety of being different? With the two cultural roles clashing? Did this reflect my fear of humiliation, transformation, and the insecurity of the changing self?

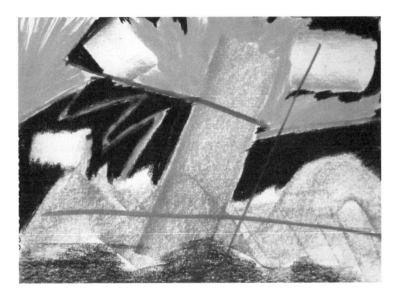

Figure 21.2 *Internal conflict and sense of inadequacy*

Entering

Pollock and Van Reken (2001) describe the stage of *entering* as entering a stage in which life is no longer so confused and muddled. "Life is no longer totally chaotic. We have made the decision that it is time to become part of this new community" (p.69). At this stage the chaos may be replaced by feelings of ambivalence. Returning to Cambridge after the Colloquium was an exhilarating experience. Each day of each week during the first year, we learned something about ourselves through the utilization of different art media: movement, music, art, journal and creative writings, or psychodrama.

Despite the self-exploration process, for the most part I remained quiet and non-expressive verbally in class and in the group process. Coming from an Eastern culture, we learn early on in our lives that expression of feelings and issues are a private matter. The Thai perception of those who share their inner selves is either "you are getting closer to being mad" (because you can't control your feelings from showing) or "you are bringing shame to your family" (because you have negative feelings or issues with them). Being assertive and speaking up for yourself, your rights, and your needs is seen as impolite and rude. Slowly through the group process, as well as the developing of trust and respect in my teachers and fellow students, I learned to accept my feelings and their importance. The concrete products of my personal artworks validated and confirmed my sense of being and feeling.

As a result, my second year was a transformative one. In my Dream Workshop with Shaun McNiff, I discovered my persona as an eagle. I learned to spread my wings and looked out with confidence with my eagle eyes. Furthermore, the integration of powerful psychodrama sessions and art therapy helped me find my voice, scream out my feelings, and celebrate who I was.

Re-involvement

Pollock and Van Reken (2001) described the last stage as:

> We may not be native to that community, but we can ultimately belong. We have learned the new ways and know our position in this community. Other members of the group see us as one of them, or at least they know where we fit in. We have a sense of intimacy, a feeling that our presence matters to this group. We feel secure. Time again feels present and permanent. (p.71)

After graduation, I remained in Massachusetts for another seven years. I was first employed by the Metropolitan State Hospital where they treated chronically mentally ill clients in a day treatment program. In addition to being an expressive therapist, I was also promoted to be the assistant director of the program for a year before I switched to being employed as an expressive therapist and a clinical supervisor at the Lawrence Schiff Day Treatment Center, a Harvard affiliated agency, and as an adjunct faculty in the Expressive Therapies Program at Lesley College Graduate School (currently Lesley University). These appointments represented the *re-involvement* stage as I developed my identity and felt grounded within the community. During my professional career in the US, I became a Registered Art Therapist (ATR), passed the board exam to become an American Board Certified Practitioner of Psychodrama (CP), a Massachusetts Licensed Mental Health Counselor (LMHC), and a Massachusetts Licensed Marriage and Family Therapist (LMFT) respectively.

Reflections on personal understanding

Looking back and reviewing my own artworks through this process of self-development, I could recall a few major shifts in my personal growth. I experienced clarity of my being in terms of my feelings, thoughts, wishes, and needs. I was able to be present in the here and now. I became more action oriented rather than awaiting my karma. I felt more grounded, validated, respected, and accepted both on a personal level as well as a professional one.

The journey did not end here. A few years after my marriage in 1995, my husband and I decided to return to Bangkok. Again I re-experienced the cycle of transitional experience. Saying goodbye to my "host country," which by then felt more like home, to go back to the "home country" was difficult and sad. Lots of questions floated around in my mind:

> Would I be able to explain to people in Thailand what art therapy and expressive therapies are? How would I be able to go forward? How could I pave the way? Would I have the opportunity to share the value of art therapy experiences? Where would I fit in?

The irony of "home coming"

May 1995, Bangkok, Thailand—soon after I got over the jet-lag, I began surveying galleries around Bangkok to see what types of art were being exhibited and tried to feel what sort of cultural reflections were being portrayed. To my dismay, the majority of "masterpieces" I encountered were heavily focused on the technical aspects of artistic skills, but from my perspective seemed to lack emotional expressions. Some were imitations of great artists of the world, but seemed to be lacking in originality. Much later, I decided to visit a university gallery. I walked in without any expectations. As I was about to exit and come around the corner, I encountered a large comical self-portrait of a young artist, Chatchai Puipia. All of his artworks portrayed the ironic side of life that could make you laugh at the naked truth and yet experienced the pain of reality at the same time. They were expressive, original, and powerful sets of oil-paintings. They exposed me to the personal and emotional expression I could not previously find, and they excited me and made me hopeful. Klausner (1993), an anthropologist who wrote his first book about Thai culture almost 40 years ago, reflected on the traditional side of that culture:

As one gingerly traverses the Thai social and cultural labyrinth, the paths chosen are curved, indirect, and circular. One avoids confrontation; one shuns direct challenge; one evades visible expression of anger, hatred, displeasure, annoyance. Conflicts are resolved through compromise. Emotional detachment and equilibrium is valued. One must not become too involved, engaged, attached. And yet, one has obligations, and duties. Emotional neutrality and distance must accommodate to the reality of "social place," one's position on the ladder of status, seniority, wealth, rank, power and prestige. One must accord proper deference, respect and diffidence towards those in more exalted positions whether it be a parent, teacher, patron, business or civil service superior. (p.386)

I thought back to the art of Chatcahi Puipia, and recognized that his works were samples of contradictions to Klausner's description and that contemporary Thai culture is undergoing tremendous transformation and change. Puipia's art was sarcastic, stark, blunt, and emotionally raw. He confronted pain in the *Siamese Smiles* (Figure 21.3) and in the *Tradition/Tensions* series (A Leg Up Society, 2010). His views portrayed the absurdity of a society by shaking it from emotional detachment and the existing state of equilibrium. Audiences were drawn to engage with his message. I saw a light at the end of the tunnel to counter the traditional Thai perceptions of mental health services as only for "crazy ones" and that "one should be ashamed and embarrassed if you break the family secrets by sharing your innermost experience with a stranger." I wanted to demonstrate that the therapeutic process can help people review, explore, and resolve issues, but also enhance personal growth to assist in reaching one's full potential.

During the first few months of my return, I thought that clinical experience abroad in addition to accredited credentials from prestige institutions would earn respect and prove my competency. I soon became disillusioned. I went for an interview looking to volunteer for clinical work and an opportunity to introduce art therapy in a day treatment program at a governmental hospital, which is also a well-respected medical school. After reading my long resumé, the very first question asked by the Head of the Department of Psychiatry was, "Do you think you will be able to understand the Thai people?" My retort: "Well, in the US where I worked professionally for seven years, my clients and my colleagues accepted me for who I was, even though I look different and have an Asian accent. I connect with people through being genuine with respect. Art therapy can be a powerful medium to help people explore and to discover who they are. The therapeutic art process can help externalize suppressed and repressed feelings. In addition, one can use art therapy assessments for diagnostic purposes and for tracking the clients' mental status as well as treatment progress." She gave me three months to do a pilot program in art therapy with the inpatient and outpatient clients who attended the day program.

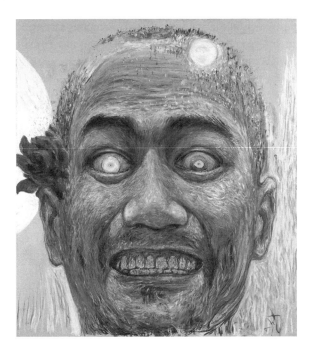

Figure 21.3 *The Siamese Smiles (by Chatchai Puipia)*

The treatment team on the unit consisted of multidisciplinary team members who seemed to be kind and open to learning about art therapy. The two main art therapy assessment tools I used at the time were Silver's (2002) Drawing Test (for an initial assessment which helped me place clients in an appropriate group according to their level of functioning and to get a glimpse of therapeutic issues) and the Diagnostic Drawing Series (Cohen, Hammer and Singer, 1988) for a mid-way assessment of progress. In addition, I used Kinetic Family Drawings (Burns and Kaufman, 1970) to assess perceptions of family and explore family dynamics (as one of the group activities). This art therapy group was an open group where we had patients from an inpatient psychiatric ward who attended the day treatment program as a part of their transition before being discharged from the ward. We also had clients who came to the program as a part of their outpatient treatment plans to help maintain stability in mental health.

In art therapy sessions, we began the group by verbally checking in to evaluate briefly their mental status; then, we moved on to the warm-up phase. Although in the first few weeks group members were a bit shy and inhibited in using art media, I introduced art warm-up activities to help reduce performance anxiety and to assist members in developing their trust and interpersonal connectedness. Structure and consistency were very important external factors to help increase internal safety with this psychiatric population. Once the therapeutic issues emerged, I assigned a topic for the group. In many situations, I utilized art interventions to help redirect clients to be more grounded, interactive with one another, and to express further their feelings through symbolism. Once emotions were being concretely represented and acknowledged, group members validated their own feelings as well as others'. Over a period of time, one could experience a few of Yalom's (1995) Therapeutic Factors such as group cohesion, installation of hope, and universality.

Despite the coming and going of members, the clients seemed to be comfortable and expressive both on the pictorial and verbal levels. During the art therapy sessions, clients responded in ways that they had not communicated through other treatment modalities. Personal and family issues were expressed, and worked on both symbolic and verbal levels. Imagery and colors created by the clients were more powerful and intense than words could describe. Instead of feeling the "cultural shame" of sharing their issues, they felt less isolated and more understood by group members. They began to experience what Yalom defines as a sense of "universality" with their peers who shared similar therapeutic themes. At rounds and case conferences, medical and clinical staff began to appreciate the value of art therapy.

During an informal conversation with the head nurse on the unit, she asked me, "Which connection did you come from?" I was a bit puzzled, but quickly regained my wit: "A telephone connection." It is generally acknowledged that to move up the social or professional hierarchy quickly in Thailand, you need a connection. As it happened, at the end of three months, a position was open for a clinician. Unfortunately, my telephone connection could not perform magic, so I left when my pilot program was completed. For a few years after this, I worked for private organizations doing clinical work and art therapy groups with primary-aged children.

Building the bridges

Little by little, art therapy began to gain its ground. The Thai Department of Mental Health contacted one of the agencies for whom I worked and requested a training workshop on the topic of art therapy for their mental health professionals, including psychiatrists, social workers, psychiatric nurses, and occupational therapists. Later, I was invited to conduct another workshop at the Department of Mental Health National Conference to demystify art therapy. These were challenging years, as the Thai view of art in clinical contexts is that it is for fun and recreation.

In order for them to experience the seriousness of the therapeutic effects in the process, I conducted my later trainings with experiential exercises and adapted some warm-up exercises that utilized culturally oriented themes, so that they could relate and identify with the symbolism represented in artworks. For example, I used several photographs of temples, different weather conditions with Thai scenes in the background, and places on Bangkok streets for them to select to represent their "state of mind" in the here and now; then they were to select another photograph to represent a "state of mind" where they wanted to be. We then worked on how to achieve their goals in concrete ways within the psychosocial model.

Other examples were "Imagine and draw a symbol of an expected role as a dutiful son/daughter of your parents versus a symbol of a role in which you want to be," or "Divide up a piece of paper into two sides. Draw how others perceive you versus how you really feel inside." Following the warm-up, the therapeutic process of opening up to share experiences followed naturally. A box of tissues became one of the essential materials in a workshop. Most of the training workshops emphasized the "process" as a way to raise awareness from the subconscious contradictions of feelings to the attentiveness of consciousness of one's needs and self-care, which also validated the importance of the self and others, as Thais have a tendency to neglect their own needs. Culturally, when one is focused on being attentive to one's own needs, the individual is viewed as being "selfish." Giving the opportunity to express, the creative art process paves the way for self-development for a fuller potential. Once these multidisciplinary staff experienced the process of the changing self and had increased their self-care, they were able to provide better mental health services to their clients.

In May 2010, two weeks after the political riot in Bangkok, I conducted a workshop to debrief people who lived near the riot sites using art therapy as a medium to explore. Themes of power struggle, corruption, and violence led workshop participants to express their senses of fear, anger, despair, and depression. As the process progressed, a sense of hope emerged from this shared experience (Figures 21.4 and 21.5). About a month after this workshop, I had an opportunity to do a follow-up with the same people in a discussion group. The participants compared their reactions after the May riot to their reactions when the tsunami hit the south of Thailand on 26 December 2004. Post-tsunami, news media bombarded the audience with visual images and horror stories. As a result, many viewers were subjected to what is called "secondary exposure" which resulted in secondary post-traumatic stress disorder. One of the workshop members stated:

> After watching so many tsunami scenes on the TV, I became depressed and felt hopeless for months. I did not speak to anyone; I thought something was wrong with me. But this time around with the political riot, I have not become depressed. I think that what we have done with the creative arts has helped. I have felt that I was not the only one who felt the rage at the rioters. The painting helped me express my dark feelings. I do not have to feel guilty for having anger.

Many members in that group agreed with her. Typically in Thai culture, when one experiences anger, one should not express nor hold on to it. Anger is viewed as bad even if it is justified. Thai Buddhists believe that you should forgive the others. If you hold on to the anger and resentment, you are then perceived as a "non-forgiver," a person who possesses grudges and lives an unhappy life. The power of expressive arts therapy, in this instance, demonstrates that the ability and opportunity to express and externalize fear and anger helps to prevent the downfall into depression, which might otherwise be a result of the traumatic incident. The therapeutic process of sharing, validating, and accepting feelings had assisted the people affected by the recent riots, to enhance and reinforce their coping strategies.

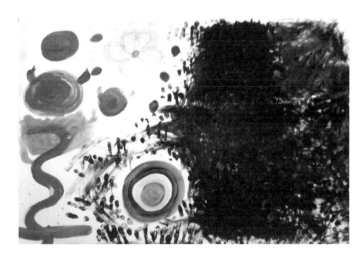

Figure 21.4 *Processing the post riot*

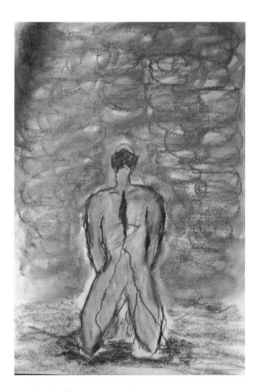

Figure 21.5 *An individual's reaction to the riot*

Conclusion

Having done a 360-degree turn around Pollock and Van Reken's transitional stages of cultural experiences helped equip me to work with Thai people who have gone abroad to study and have returned home, as well as with those non-Thais who came to Thailand as a "host country," who experienced culture shock. On the professional level, I feel as if I have once again entered the "re-involvement" stage on the Third Culture Kids model. Over the years of hard working and believing in the power of the therapeutic process of expressive arts therapy, I have gained respect from professionals from various disciplines. As an example, art therapy has made its way to court rooms. The Ministry of Justice has chosen this modality as one of the core treatments in the Juvenile Detention Centers all over the nation. Ongoing training in art therapy for the counselors of the Youth Correctional System has been organized on a regular basis. A few of my clients' work have been used as evidence to testify in their court cases. As for the Ministry of Education, they have organized many events in which "art for self and social development" has been used to promote children's emotional intelligence (EQ), and many school summer camps have incorporated "art for self-exploration" in their programs.

On a personal level, I feel that I am at the point where I can appreciate and have empathy for those who experience cultural struggles. For the first seven years of my return here, I was stuck in the process of trying to prove that the Western ways might have been better, but now I feel as if I can integrate the two worlds of the East and the West into my understanding of myself and others. There are merits in Thai culture that should be acknowledged. For example, the concept of being in the "here and now" was taken from Eastern philosophy. It is an example of a balanced integration. "To be present" also helps one be attentive to what's going on with the self on all levels whether it be physical, emotional, or spiritual. Paying attention to self-care is a Western concept, which at times may come across to the Eastern perception as being self-centered or selfish. However, when you put these two concepts together, the "here and now" and "self-care," both sides of the cultural opposite can understand them in a non-abrasive manner. For me, this example represents a journey of integration that has led me to a meaningful practice of art therapy in Thailand.

References

A Leg Up Society (2010) *Chatchai is Dead, If Not, He Should Be.* Bangkok, Thailand: Amarin Printing and Publishing Public Company.

Burns, R. and Kaufman, S.H. (1970) *Kinetic Family Drawings (K-F-D): An Introduction to Understanding Children through Kinetic Drawings.* New York, NY: Brunner/Mazel.

Cohen, B.M., Hammer, J.S. and Singer, S. (1988) "The Diagnostic Drawing Series: A systematic approach to art therapy evaluation and research." *The Arts in Psychotherapy 15,* 1, 11–21.

Klausner, W.J. (1993) *Reflections on Thai Culture.* Bangkok, Thailand: The Siam Society.

Pollock, D.C. and Van Reken, R.E. (2001) *Third Culture Kids: The Experience of Growing Up Among Worlds.* Boston, MA: Nicholas Brealey Publishing.

Silver, R. (2002) *Three Art Assessment.* New York, NY: Brunner-Routledge.

Yalom, I.D. (1995) *Theory and Practice of Group Psychotherapy.* New York, NY: Basic Books.

Chapter 22

Implications of Art Therapy in Asia

Debra Kalmanowitz, Jordan S. Potash and Siu Mei Chan

One of the lingering questions that pervades the experience of this book is, 'What does it mean to have an Asian model of art therapy and is it necessary or important?' This book began with the intention of documenting the range of art therapy practices throughout Asia in order to determine how they relate to specific cultural ideas and values. While the six themes around which this book has been organized potentially provide a context for a model, in this final chapter we hope to distil emerging ideas on possible tensions, features and variations, as well as how these ideas can affect not only the practice of art therapy in Asia, but also around the globe.

Traditional and the modern

Throughout the world people are looking to pave the way for a more just, improved and peaceful way of living and being. Throughout the world people are looking for cures to illness and the key to living a harmonious balanced life, a life which provides health and prosperity, quality and wellbeing. Progress is taken as essential for sustainable development, environmental protection, improvement in health, both of adults and children, and to a certain degree participation in democratic social and political processes. Conflict between the new and the old, the traditional and the modern, are strong undercurrents that move people's motivation into an emotional easiness or uneasiness of which they may not even be aware. The backdrop of this book is the struggle or the balance between two worlds, and the new and the old are represented to a different degree in every chapter.

Phillips and James (2001) address this contradiction between traditional and 'modernisation', as they refer to it. They argue against identity as being one-dimensional and instead put forward the idea that emphasizes the contradictory layering of identity. Their article deconstructs the notion that the formation of identity involves the termination of traditional ties. Rather, they suggest that a layering of subjective experiences is likely to continue which leaves the individuals caught in a series of tensions between traditionalism and modernization. They continue that the myth of modernity is that it cancels all before it, turning the traditional way of life into mere fragments to be used by what they call 'carriers' to build a nation. This debate is one in which it is important for us to engage in this book. What we have found does indeed mirror these sentiments. The models and styles of work created across Asia are multi-layered. An understanding which polarizes the two ends of the spectrum leads to a simplified and stereotypical understanding of the subject, a stance of which we caution against.

By shifting the conversation from tradition vs. contemporary to tradition and contemporary, we can arrive at a middle ground. The intention is not to judge, but to reflect upon the different choices individuals make and the impact these choices have on art therapy models and practices. There is no right or wrong, good or bad. We all work within our own bounds, but we believe that it is possible to say that there is an Asian style, which has much to contribute to the world, and already does.

Change is taking place. Whether we like it or not things change, as there is a natural push to progress in whatever form this takes. The question is what we do with the change. Do we drag it through the mud or do we accept it in the spirit of keeping the peace that the traditional world was trying to preserve? Indeed, there is no such thing as a static culture. Change is continual, and flexibility is necessary for successful adaptation. Indeed it seems that change and consistency or stability live side by side. It is not either/or, but it is in fact the yin and yang, the balance we all seek and that is so integral to Asian thinking. To some degree we all try to balance these forces to create a life and a work which has meaning. Art therapy is no exception, and neither is art therapy in Asia.

Tensions in Asian art therapy

Although not explicitly described within the chapters themselves, there are tensions that we noticed as a result of our interaction with authors and in conversations with others about the nature and necessity of this book. We feel these tensions are worth noting not only as they relate specifically to Asia, but also as they have relevance for the development of art therapy across the world in general.

Bone vs. silk

Relating back to the comment made by our colleague that was referenced in Chapter 1, we have tried to tease out if art therapy in Asia is truly unique or if it only has a distinct local costume that makes it more familiar. The range of practices in this book show both. Although one might think that having a fundamentally Asian core (bone) would make the practice more authentic, some of the chapters demonstrate how providing themes and culturally relevant interpretations (silk) allows the practice to be effective.

Romantic vs. everyday

In compiling, researching and reflecting on this book, we realized that beyond documentation we were looking for differences in the way that art therapy is practised in Asia. Although differences are present and real (as are similarities and overlaps), we are aware that the shadow side of looking for difference is a potential to romanticize or perhaps even idealize the other. This tendency is as much a cultural blindness as ignoring unique cultural values. This point is important to consider when reflecting on the role of culture in forming new models. As Asia moves onto the world stage and its philosophies are embraced by the West, we are particularly cautious of over-simplifying the theories we are discussing and careful to see them within their broader context.

Distinct vs. universal

Similar to the previous challenge, there is a tension between wanting to show that the practices in Asia are not all that different from those in the West, but at the same time wanting to show distinctions. It could be that the wanting to be similar is a representation of embracing contemporary thinking, while the highlighting of culture is a way to show pride in heritage and the limits of simply importing practices. This tension also seems to relate to the fact that despite being aware of cultural influences and the existence of traditional ideas, not everyone in a given society or culture bases their work on these ideas. For example, the two examples of using Traditional Chinese Medicine (Gong in Chapter 3, as well as Richardson, Gollub and Wang in Chapter 4), while showing how those specific practitioners work, are not indications of how all art therapists work across China.

Intentional vs. interpretation

It was at times unclear if cultural values were instilled in the models from the outset or if they were used as a frame for review in retrospect. While interpretation can be helpful in making meaning, instituting interpretations after the fact is quite different to it being an innate and integral part of the working model. This observation, however, is not to say that one is better or more desirable than the other. While the intentional ensures the building of a culturally relevant model, the interpretation allows for a culturally relevant understanding of art therapy practice. Both are necessary for the acceptance and integration of art therapy throughout Asia.

Cultural blindness vs. cultural irrelevance

Given the scope of the book to document practices with specific reference to how they have been integrated and adapted throughout Asia, we often encouraged authors to return to their practice to identify values and ideas that made their work unique in the countries in which they were working. It was not always obvious where culture or cultural adaptations had been made, or if they fit at all. There were times when we were forced to question and re-question ourselves, our own framework of understanding, and where we fit into this continuum. As the book, our research and thinking has progressed, however, we have become more and more clear that culture permeates all aspects of life (overtly or covertly, conscious or unconscious), so the idea that it would not have an impact to a greater or lesser degree seems absurd. What the experience has taught us, however, is that, when culture is ever present, it can be difficult to see, much like the fish who does not see the water until it is removed from it.

Features of a developing art therapy

Interestingly then, what emerges is a notion of a possible model which is relevant across the globe and significant and pertinent to Asia, but not necessarily specific to it. This of course is taking into account the ability to balance the cultural specifics and significance (as discussed in Chapter 2) with the general principles and understanding (as discussed in this chapter).

Takes into account cultural values

As is evident, what has emerged as a most palpable concern is the degree to which culture plays a part, whether it be explicitly or implicitly. Clearly, cultural values can help guide and shape an art therapy practice, but are not necessarily at the forefront of the work. For the authors in this book, these values shaped first and foremost the way in which they related to their clients, and the families of the clients. At times this interaction may be where the influence stopped, while at other times it served to fashion the theoretical framework, treatment goals and service delivery. In terms of practice, values guided themes, directives, structure, and interpretation. The examples shared by Byrne in her work with senior adults in Hong Kong (Chapter 8), and Alfonso and Byers in their relief work in the Philippines (Chapter 19), reveal a sensitivity to the important value of interpersonal relationships within a family and society. This same sensitivity was role modelled by Tan (Chapter 20) in creating a group process that directly benefits her clients in Cambodia while instigating change on a societal level. Sezaki's observations (Chapter 16) on the importance of hierarchy in the client–therapist relationship influenced his decision on the level of structure that he offers in his groups in Japan. Similarly, Essame's protocols (Chapter 6) offer culturally infused guidelines for art therapy practice.

Takes into consideration local ideas of art

Another feature is the influence and integration of traditional ideas on art. Western art therapy is directly influenced by art history in Europe and the United States, so it is not surprising that the art history in each country of Asia would shape its art therapy practice. Liang's and Singh's descriptions of art in China and India respectively (Chapters 12 and 13) indicate historical accounts of using the arts to achieve balance and harmony within an individual. In this sense, the influence on art therapy is not just in the fact that art can express something, but that art can perform the important role of stabilization and equilibrium. Although the book was conceived as art therapy – that is, visual art – we can see the continuum of and integration of the arts that permeated many of the chapters. Whether Chang's intentional use of the expressive arts (Chapter 18) or Herbert's spontaneous use of music and dance (Chapter 15), the art forms while offering their own unique benefits may not have the artificial separation that is often the norm in the West.

Takes into consideration indigenous ideas of therapy, healing and medicine

In both obvious and unobvious ways, traditional ideas on health become infused with art therapy practice. The examples of Traditional Chinese Medicine offered by Richardson, Gollub and Wang, as well as by Gong, demonstrate an intentional integration of these ideas. The difference, of course, is that Wang saw the benefit of bringing art into traditional medicine, whereas Gong learned the benefit of bringing Traditional Chinese Medicine into her art therapy. Still, in both examples, the integration of these ideas are core to their work. In their own ways, Pluckpankhajee's and Chua's explorations (Chapters 9 and 10) demonstrate the long-standing healing practices associated with Buddhism and how they can inform and enhance art therapy.

Integrates what works and adapts what does not

Another feature seems to be looking at the practice of art therapy in relation to the West. This statement is not to say that the West is the standard and Asia is a derivative, but rather in the recognition that there are two developing ideas. While there is overlap, there are differences. This idea is highlighted by the fact that there are more art therapists working in Asia who are trained in the West than there are Western art therapists trained in Asia. As a result, Asian-based art therapists have to make decisions as to what to take in from the West and what to let go. Lee's example (Chapter 7) demonstrates the limits of individual focus that are so important in Western art therapy literature, yet still demonstrates recognition of its value, so long as it is not at the expense of the family. Perhaps in a less obvious way, Lu (Chapter 17) shared a model that demonstrates the importance of researching the appropriateness of applying a Western framework (in her case, Lowenfeld's art development stages). Rappaport, Ikemi and Miyake (Chapter 11) additionally show the need to infuse a Western practice with mindfulness to mirror expectations in Japan, while Katmonowitz and Potash (Chapter 14) demonstrate the necessity to modify both theory and practice in China. Making these decisions provides new ways to re-conceptualize art therapy for use throughout the region and in other parts of the world. As Kim suggested (Chapter 5), the integration and knowing when to make use of theories from around the globe points to a more informed health practice.

Re-imagining art therapy

There is sometimes a tendency to focus on how the West has influenced the rest of the world, but a more scholarly look at history reveals that when cultures meet they mutually influence each other. Art history in the West took a radical turn in the mid-19th century with the rise of the Impressionists and Post-Impressionists. Although technological and industrial advances played roles in ushering in this new art tradition, Kleiner and Mamiya (2005) point to the introduction of Japanese culture to Western artists. We only need to look at Monet's creation of a Japanese-style garden at his studio home in Giverny with the resulting iconic paintings of water lilies and the new compositional elements utilized by other artists such as Degas, Cassat, Van Gogh and Gauguin. The two-dimensional spaces and the patterned decorative elements evident in Japanese woodblock prints were borrowed by these artists as they found new ways to depict space, represent patterns and include areas of flat colour in their drawings and paintings. Japanese artistic inclusion of decorative elements and aesthetic attention paid to utilitarian objects also influenced the artists of the Art Nouveau and the Arts and Crafts movement. Images and artists we view as essential and quintessential to Western art history as well as all the artists that followed them can trace their origins in part to Asia.

As in art, the same trend can be traced in therapy. Kabat-Zinn (1994), a student of Zen master Seung Sahn, brought yoga and meditation to the practice of psychology in the West. He teaches mindfulness meditation to help people cope with stress, anxiety, pain and illness. Kabat-Zinn fits into a stream of Western psychological approaches that draw on the ideas of mindfulness and the connection between the body and the mind. Acceptance commitment therapy (ACT) uses acceptance and mindfulness strategies, along with behaviour strategies, to encourage psychological flexibility (Hayes, Strosahl and Wilson, 1999). Dialectical behaviour therapy (DBT) combines cognitive behavioural techniques with mindfulness in treatment (Linehan, 1995). In addition to combining the Western behavioural techniques with mindfulness, she also draws on the ideas of the Vietnamese Buddhist monk Thich Nhat Hanh in creating a climate of unconditional acceptance.

In addition to these approaches, there are numerous treatment methods in the West today that are inspired by Asian practices. Energy psychology addresses the relationship of energy systems to emotion, cognition, behaviour and health. The understanding is that psychological functioning involves an essential level of bioenergy. The energy diagnostic and treatment method (EDXTM), developed by Gallo (1998), describes a diagnostic system based on energy psychology and uses diagnostic treatments rooted in an energy paradigm. In this technique, Gallo takes into account energy approaches such as working with the meridians as in acupuncture and kinesiology.

Somatic psychology is an interdisciplinary field involving the study of the mind and our somatic experiences, our experiences in the body or embodied experiences. This is considered a holistic approach to the body and is a field of study that tries to bridge the mind–body dichotomy. Although these specific therapies in the West can trace their origins back to Wilhelm Reich (Sharaf, 1983), the first psychotherapist to bring body awareness into psychotherapy, there is an increasing use of body-oriented techniques within mainstream psychology today. The use of mindfulness, eye movement desensitization and reprocessing (EMDR) and psychoanalysis itself has for some years recognized the somatic significance or reverberations of trauma, for example. This is of course reminiscent of the holistic approach to the mind and body we have discussed throughout the book, and indeed this revisiting of the mind–body dichotomy in a Western context can credit the dialogue between the East and the West and the opening up of consciousness on both sides of the world to embrace philosophies and ideas that can contribute to existing systems, whatever they are and wherever they begin.

Just as all of these individuals learned from Asia and incorporated the ideas into Western practice, so too have we seen that art therapists from Asia learn from their colleagues across the globe. The art therapy practices explored in this book represent an art therapy that is not limited to the exploration of individual consciousness or narrowly focused on clinical models. By incorporating the wisdom and applications of art therapy in the West and Asia into the global discourse, we can imagine a practice of art therapy categorized as much by art therapy for meditation, prevention and holistic health, as well as art therapy for diagnostics, analysis and treatment.

This idea leads us back to our question, 'Asian to the bone or wrapped in silk?' The desire to create order and to find meaning, where it is not yet clear, is not specific to any one culture and in fact runs across all cultures. Although it may be tempting to superimpose practices from one culture to another, from Asia to the West or vice versa, we must be attentive not to simply apply a logic which is external to our way of thinking. When ideas emerge from a culture and find resonance with another one, a newly developed awareness can form; not one imposed, but one that grows through the combination of innate ideas and outside inspiration. To maintain integrity, art therapy globally needs to maintain its links to its roots in health, the arts and the culture in which it is practised and from which it comes.

Limitations

There are obvious limitations to this volume that are worth noting. One of the greatest is limited accessibility to practitioners working throughout Asia. Currently, there is no single association or networking group to connect art therapists in Asia or even in individual countries. With the publication of this book and development of technology, we hope that interconnectivity will grow. At times we believe that the lack of interconnectivity may have contributed to some of the authors' inability to access contemporary theories, books, journals and art therapy literature, which would have enabled them to contextualize their work within a bigger picture. We are also aware that there is a bias towards South East Asia and that there are countries in Asia that are not represented in the book despite having art therapists working in their systems. India, for example, is not amply represented. This loss is significant as the Hindu philosophy, Indian arts and Ayurveda perspective is important in this region given its impact on many neighbouring countries. Lastly, while choosing to work in English provided a universal platform among the diverse languages of Asia, we know that there are resources written in the local tongue of each area and that only individuals of particular education levels will be able to make use of this book. As we see this book as a beginning and not an end, we hope that others will join us in further identifying, documenting and disseminating the important contributions of art therapy in Asia.

Conclusion

This book has followed a path of exploration. It has brought together as many authors as was possible working in art therapy in Asia at the moment of writing. We hope that by placing these chapters together in one volume we are contributing to the expansion of thinking and global practice of art therapy. We hope that, while focusing on Asia specifically, we have succeeded in expanding the view of art therapy as a whole, and that we contribute our voice to the dialogue between the East and the West.

References

Gallo, F.P. (1998) *Energy Psychology*. New York, NY: CRC Press.

Hayes, S.C., Strosahl, K.D. and Wilson, K.G. (1999) *Acceptance and Commitment Therapy: An Experiential Approach to Behavioral Change*. New York, NY: Guilford Press.

Kabat-Zinn, J. (1994) *Wherever You Go, There You Are: Mindfulness Meditation for Every Day*. London: Piatkus.

Kleiner, F.S. and Mamiya, C.J. (2005) *Gardner's Art Through the Ages: Vol. 2*, 12th edn. Belmont, CA: Wadsworth/Thomson Learning.

Linehan, M.M. (1995) *Understanding Borderline Personality Disorder: The Dialectic Approach Program Manual*. New York, NY: Guilford Press.

Phillips, A. and James, P. (2001) 'National identity between tradition and reflexive modernisation: The contradictions of Central Asia.' *National Identities 3*, 1, 23–34.

Sharaf, M. (1983) *Fury on Earth*. New York, NY: St. Martin's Press/Marek.

Contributors

It is traditional in Asia to write one's surname (or family name) followed by the given name. The contributors list is organized alphabetically by surname (which is capitalized), but the order of the names for each of the contributors appears according to their preference.

Gina A. ALFONSO, MS Ed, MA, ATR, born and raised in the Philippines, currently resides in Washington DC, USA, where she works as an expressive arts therapist and education/art therapy consultant. She completed an MS Ed from Fordham University and an MA in Art Therapy from Lesley University. She is the founder of Cartwheel Foundation, Inc. and is pursuing a doctorate in Expressive Therapies at the European Graduate School.

Julia Gentleman BYERS, EdD, LMHC, ATR-BC, is currently the Coordinator of Graduate Studies in Art Therapy, Co-coordinator of the Advanced Professional Certificate in Play Therapy, and PhD Senior Advisor in the PhD programmes in Educational Interdisciplinary Studies and Expressive Therapies at Lesley University, Cambridge, MA, USA. She has provided professional training, consulting, workshops, disaster interventions and lectures in over 14 countries.

Julia BYRNE, MA, grew up in Hong Kong and holds a masters degree in Art Therapy/Art Education from Florida State University (1994). She has extensive experience piloting art therapy programmes in local NGOs; client groups include depression, schizophrenia, autism and ADHD, geriatrics, rehabilitation, substance abusers, domestic violence and trauma survivors. Julia is the founding president of the Hong Kong Association of Art Therapists.

Siu Mei CHAN, MA, RSW, is a registered art therapist (UK) and registered social worker (Hong Kong). She completed her social work training in Hong Kong and her art therapy training at Goldsmiths College, University of London. She specializes in working with children and families. She currently works at the Boys' and Girls' Clubs Association of Hong Kong and is the Treasurer and Vice Chairman of the Hong Kong Association of Art Therapists.

Fiona CHANG, MSocSc, RSW, REAT, has for the past 18 years practised integrated multimodal arts in a variety of settings. She is the Vice-Chairperson of 'Art in Hospital', Honorary Lecturer at the University of Hong Kong, and advisor of Art Therapy Without Borders at Southwestern College in Santa Fe. She is interested in blending Chinese metaphors and a person-centred approach in arts therapy.

Yen CHUA, MA, is an artist, art therapist and educator practising in Singapore.

Caroline ESSAME, BSc, PG Dip, is a British occupational therapist and art therapist with 26 years' experience in mental health, special needs and early childhood. She has worked in Asia for 13 years in Malaysia, Hong Kong and India and currently lives in Singapore, where she developed the Masters in Art Therapy at LASALLE-SIA College of the Arts in 2005. She is now a director of a creative arts training and therapy company.

Piyachat Ruengvisesh FINNEY, MA, LMFT, LMHC, ATR, CP, is a director of SAISILP: The Centre for Creative Growth and Professional Training. She completed her BS in Education and MA in Expressive Therapies at Lesley College Graduate School, Massachusetts, USA. Currently she works in Thailand specializing in family therapy and cross-cultural issues and works with children utilizing art therapy, psychodrama and play/puppet therapy.

Andrea GOLLUB, MEd, ATR-BC, is an art therapist who has worked for 30 years with adults, adolescents and children with a multitude of diagnoses including psychosis, PTSD, DID and bipolar disorder. She currently works at Cedars Sinai Medical Center in their Share and Care early intervention programme. She believes in the ability of artistic expression as a means of healing and gaining insight. Presenting in China only increased her belief that art heals.

GONG Shu, PhD, ATR, TEP, LCSW, is an internationally acclaimed psychotherapist and director of the International *Yi Shu* Expressive Arts Healing Research Center, Soochow University, Suzhou, China. Among her many strengths are her diverse cultural background and her rich and varied educational experiences. Her unique therapeutic process is published in the book *Yi Shu: The Art of Living with Change. Integrating Traditional Chinese Medicine, Psychodrama and the Creative Arts.*

Carrie HERBERT, PGCE, is a registered member of the UK Council for Psychotherapy and the Co-Director of Arts Therapy Services for the Ragamuffin Project (INGO) in Cambodia. She is an arts psychotherapist, trainer and supervisor with extensive experience with refugees, mental health, trauma and abuse, post conflict and emergencies, therapeutic training, and clinical and organizational supervision. As an international consultant, she has worked in India, Singapore, Indonesia, Hong Kong and Peru.

Akira IKEMI Ph.D. is a professor of clinical psychology at Kansai University Graduate School of Professional Clinical Psychology. He is a board member of the Focusing Institute (NY) and former president of the Japan Focusing Association. He practices Focusing-Oriented Psychotherapy and has written numerous books and articles on the subject.

Debra KALMANOWITZ, MA, RATh, is a Registered Art Therapist (UK), a Research Postgraduate, Department of Social Work and Social Administration and Honorary Clinical Associate, Centre on Behavioral Health University of Hong Kong. She has worked extensively in the context of trauma, political violence, and social change. Debra is the co-author of *The Portable Studio: art therapy and political conflict: Initiatives in the former Yugoslavia and South Africa* and the edited book *Art Therapy and Political Violence: With art, without illusion*.

Sun Hyun KIM, PhD, is Assistant Professor in Clinical Art Therapy at the Graduate School of Complementary Alternative Medicine in Pochon CHA University. She is also Director of the Art Therapy Clinic, CHA Biomedical Center, Pochon CHA University and Research Institute of East–West Art Therapy. She is a President of the Korean Academy of Clinical Art Therapy as well as Beijing, Seoul, Tokyo Association of Clinical Art Therapy (BESETO CAT).

LEE Min Jung, MA, completed a BA in Special Education at Ewha Woman's University (Seoul, Korea) and MA in Creative Arts Therapy at Hofstra University (New York, USA). She is currently working as an art therapist at the Seocho Institute for Child Development (Seoul, Korea) and as a lecturer at the Korean Academy of Clinical Art Therapy (Seoul, Korea).

Evelyna LIANG Kan, DFA, has worked for the past 40 years as an artist, art educator and community artist in needy and underprivileged communities using her community art model. Evelyna has exhibited extensively in Hong Kong and Asia. Her interest has extended into the area of 'Healing through Art' using ordinary daily objects to explore the relationship between different people and countries.

Liona LU, DFA, ATR-BC, has been Professor in the Department of Visual Arts and Graduate Art Therapy Program in Taipei Municipal University of Education (TMUE) since 1989. In 2004, she founded the Taiwan Art Therapy Association, and in the following year she founded the art therapy programme in TMUE. Currently, she has a part-time practice in the Taiwan Institute of Psychotherapy, where she works with children, adults and families.

Maki MIYAKE, Ph.D. is a Certified Clinical Psychologist and a Focusing Institute Trainer. She is an adjunct faculty member at Kansai University and at Osaka University of Economics. Maki Miyake practices psychotherapy in a private practice and at an automobile corporation in Japan.

Anupan PLUCKPANKHAJEE, DipAT, studied Anthroposophical Art Therapy in Germany. He has worked for UNODC and the Bureau of Anti-Human Trafficking and has used art therapy as a treatment in hospital by focusing on emotional problems. Currently, Anupan works as an artist and is the director of the Therapeutikum (Thailand).

Jordan S. POTASH, PhD, ATR-BC, LCAT, is a Teaching Consultant and Expressive Arts Therapy Coordinator for the Centre on Behavioral Health, University of Hong Kong. Interested in social change, he promotes art therapy for reducing stigma, confronting discrimination and promoting cross-cultural relationships. He was chair of the Multicultural Committee, American Art Therapy Association, and is the Book Review Editor for *Art Therapy: Journal of the American Art Therapy Association*.

Laury RAPPAPORT, Ph.D., ATR-BC, REAT is an Associate Professor at Notre Dame de Namur University and taught at Lesley University for over 30 years. She is a Focusing Coordinator with The Focusing Institute, the Founder/Director of the Focusing and Expressive Arts institute, on the Advisory Board of Art Therapy without Borders, and the author of *Focusing-Oriented Art Therapy*.

Jane Ferris RICHARDSON, EdD, ATR-BC, RPT-S, is an art therapist and core faculty member at Lesley University. She also exhibits her artwork regularly. Her private practice specializes in children and special needs. Her research interests include the arts and autism. Jane has presented her work internationally, travelling with colleagues to China and Japan, and, most recently, with students to Cape Town, South Africa.

Shinya SEZAKI, MA, is an art therapist working with adult psychiatric patients at Akimoto Hospital, in Chiba, Japan. He is a lecturer at Tokyo Zokei University and the author of a comprehensive guide to group art therapy in Japan. He has previously published in *Art Therapy: Journal of the American Art Therapy Association.*

Shanta Serbjeet SINGH is a senior arts columnist and critic, author of several books on Indian dance and music, and is the elected Chairperson of India's national cultural body (the Sangeet Natak Akademi) and of the Asia-Pacific Performing Arts Network, set up under the aegis of UNESCO.

Lydia Atira TAN, DipAT, is an expressive art therapist, visual artist and yoga and meditation teacher. She is the director and founder of the Art2Healing Project, an Australian non-profit organization dedicated to supporting marginalized women and children in Asia and the Pacific through creative art therapies, yoga and meditation. Lydia is dedicated to the healing of trauma in sex trafficking survivors internationally.

WANG Chunhong, a dance therapist trained in DaoYin and TuiNa massage, is Director of the Chinese Art Medicine Association. She ran groups at psychiatric hospitals and is the Director of the God Gifted Garden Art Rehabilitation Center, where she uses a unique combination of dance, music and art combined with theories from Chinese medicine which she calls Dimensionalartdance (DaDance).

Subject Index

Author Index